Living with
Spina Bifida

Living with

Spina Bifida

A Guide for Families
and Professionals

ADRIAN SANDLER, M.D.

Illustrations by Peter Bedick

With a New Preface by the Author

The University of North Carolina Press

Chapel Hill and London

© 1997 The University of North
Carolina Press
Preface © 2004 The University of
North Carolina Press
All rights reserved
Manufactured in the United States of
America

The paper in this book meets the guidelines
for permanence and durability of the
Committee on Production Guidelines for
Book Longevity of the Council on Library
Resources.

The Library of Congress has cataloged the
original edition of this book as follows:

Sandler, Adrian.
    Living with spina bifida : a guide for fami-
lies and professionals / by Adrian Sandler ;
illustrations by Peter Bedick.
        p.   cm.
    Includes index.
    1. Spina bifida.   2. Spina bifida—
Patients—Rehabilitation.   I. Title.
RJ496.S74S26   1997
618.92'83—dc21   96-47697
                                          CIP

ISBN 0-8078-5547-2 (pbk.)

08 07 06 05 04   5 4 3 2 1

Adrian Sandler, M.D., a native of Zimbabwe,
was educated at the University of
Cambridge, England, where he earned his
undergraduate degrees and then, in 1982, his
medical degree. He did his pediatrics resi-
dency at Duke University Medical Center
and then completed a three-year fellowship
program in developmental pediatrics at the
University of North Carolina at Chapel Hill.
Dr. Sandler was on the full-time academic
staff in the Department of Pediatrics at UNC
until 1994. Since then, he has been the medical
director of the Olson Huff Center at Mission
Children's Hospital in Asheville, North
Carolina, a busy regional center serving
children with special needs.

To Shirley,

whose support and encouragement never wavered

Contents

Preface

The field of spina bifida is going through exciting times—in clinical information, in scientific research, and in policy. Although this book, first published in 1997, remains current, I thought it important to rewrite the preface, highlighting these important areas of progress and some of the challenges that lie ahead.

The Americans with Disabilities Act (ADA), signed into law in 1992, firmly established the rights of people with disabilities and will continue to have a profound effect on American society. Similar progress has been made in many other countries around the world. Environmental barriers affect the health and well-being of people with disabilities, and compliance with the ADA will help overcome some of these barriers in schools, in the workplace, and in the community. The U.S. government's roadmap for a national health policy, entitled Healthy People 2010, sets several key objectives for promoting the health of people with disabilities, preventing secondary conditions, and eliminating disparities between people with and without disabilities.

For children with spina bifida and their families, access to affordable health care is critical. This may be especially important in the early childhood years and at times of transition to school age and young adulthood. In these times of rising health care costs, it has become increasingly difficult to fund well-coordinated, multidisciplinary spina bifida clinics, such as the one I used to direct in Chapel Hill, North Carolina. Consequently, care for thousands of children and adolescents has become more fragmented and of poorer quality. Sadly, the end result is often poorer health, more disability, and higher health care costs. We in the United States need to do better in providing access to comprehensive, coordinated health care, especially for children with special needs.

Recognizing this need, advocates and lobbyists, including those from the Spina Bifida Association of America (SBAA), have worked very hard in recent years to secure funding for prevention and for improving the quality of life of those living with spina bifida. In 2003, Congress allocated $2 million for a National Spina Bifida Program at the Centers for Disease Control and Prevention's National Center for Birth Defects and Developmental Disabilities (www.cdc.gov/ncbddd).

In May 2003, I was privileged to attend a national meeting convened by the U.S. Department of Health and Human Services to develop a research agenda, bringing together experts from medicine, surgery, and other disciplines to discuss key issues and questions related to spina bifida. A vast amount of research was reviewed, and critical priorities for further research were highlighted. The results of the meeting will help to serve as a roadmap to scientists and funding agencies in the years to come.

The first question I had to answer in writing this book regarded my audience: for whom is this book to be written? Had I written it fifteen years ago, I would have selected a limited and homogeneous group of readers. I might have written a book about spina bifida for parents of a child with this condition; or perhaps I might have written a very different book for physicians who had a special interest in the field. In the 1990s, however, when so many barriers were being broken down, it was fitting to aim the book at a wider and more inclusive readership. My perspective as a developmental-behavioral pediatrician has been greatly influenced by two interrelated models of care, namely, interdisciplinary communication and partnerships between professionals and parents (and their children too). It has become critical for professionals in different disciplines to communicate effectively, to share a certain body of knowledge and work together cooperatively for the benefit of the whole child. This has long been the case, of course, but our pursuit of expertise in ever more narrow areas of subspecialization served to isolate neurosurgeons from psychologists, orthopedic surgeons from teachers, pediatricians from physical therapists, and so on. Interdisciplinary communication has enhanced our knowledge of the field of developmental disabilities and stimulated cross-fertilization of ideas regarding management of problems and enhancement of function. Simply put, kids do better when different experts work together in a cooperative and coordinated fashion. It is also self-evident that kids do better when their parents (and they themselves) are in partnership with the different professionals caring for them, when they share similar goals and priorities and work together to develop plans of how best to achieve these goals. For a child with spina bifida to be all that she can be in life, she, her family, her teachers, her doctors, and her therapists will all be actively involved. It is in this belief that I am writing for a wide audience.

First and foremost, I am addressing the parents of children with spina bifida. The book contains most of the medical information that they will need to understand their child's condition and to participate actively in their child's health care. Relatedly, it has become increasingly evident to me in my clinical work with children and adolescents with spina bifida that their own education about spina bifida is often overlooked. I am often surprised to find that articulate young adults with spina bifida know so little about the nature of spina bifida or certain aspects of their health care. It is as if these areas are out of bounds and were not spoken about openly in their formative years. Independence and self-care depend on self-knowledge.

The book is also written for pediatricians, family physicians, and other generalists who provide health care for children, adolescents, and adults with spina bifida. Spina bifida remains the most common complex birth defect, and most general practitioners will have a few affected individuals in their practices. The management of spina bifida has undergone profound changes in the last twenty years, and many physicians may be unfamiliar with more recent management options. The "Medical Home" for children with chronic conditions such as spina bifida is usually the community pediatrician or family practitioner. Visits to specialized spina bifida clinics or to specialists' offices may be sporadic and infrequent. This book also aims, therefore, to help bridge the gap between hospital clinic and community-based care.

The book is broad in scope and contains information about diverse issues related to spina bifida that may also be of interest to specialist physicians, such as orthopedic surgeons, neurosurgeons, and urologists, who are seeking information that is outside their particular domain of expertise. As in other advancing fields of medicine, there is no single standard management for spina bifida, and different centers may employ different methods of care. Many treatment options are controversial and in the early stages of their evolution. I have attempted to provide a balanced and up-to-date account of such matters, and I obtained input from many experts, to whom I am very grateful.

Clinicians and therapists in the allied health professions, including nurses, physical therapists, occupational therapists, speech/language therapists, and nutritionists, who provide therapeutic services for individuals with spina bifida will, I hope, benefit from reading a book such as this. Also, community professionals, including psychologists and social workers, who are especially concerned with developmental, mental health, and family issues in the context of spina bifida will find this book helpful. Tertiary centers that provide subspecialty care almost invariably see affected individuals sporadically, perhaps once or twice a year, and are critically dependent on therapists in the community to carry out treatment regimens, evaluate progress, and remain vigilant for new problems.

As more and more children with spina bifida attend "regular" classes in school, the field of education (both "regular" and "special" education) must shoulder the responsibility of understanding and meeting the diverse special needs of this population. Teachers and school psychologists, who must daily confront the educational and emotional impacts of spina bifida, will find much within this book that is especially relevant to their challenges. Similarly, the issues faced by those who are concerned with postsecondary education, vocational readiness, and transitions to independent adulthood are addressed herein.

Many people advised me against attempting to bring such diverse readerships together in one book. I am committed to the idea in principle, but I recognize the difficulties and drawbacks of trying to convey that which is interesting and relevant to all. Clearly, it would be helpful to have some means of prioritizing information, recognizing that some issues are primarily of importance to parents, and perhaps secondarily of interest to doctors and other health care professionals. Other matters may be particularly relevant for psychologists and educators, and so on. To assist the reader, I have highlighted areas in the text that I feel are specially written for one audience or another with color codes. Highly technical sections written in "medicalese" are marked with a black band in the margin. Sections that are specifically addressed to parents carry a red band. These should serve only as a guide, and I hope that most readers, irrespective of their discipline, will find the entire book relevant and easy to read. As the reader will see, most of the book is not color coded, reflecting my bias that, for the most part, the content of the book crosses boundaries. A glossary of terms that are frequently used is included.

Chapter 1 provides a holistic overview of the condition of spina bifida and touches on some of the themes that run through the book. The brief clinical overview of spina bifida given here may suffice for the reader who does not want to venture into more detailed information about the medical aspects of the condition. Important issues in the normal development of children and adolescents are introduced as we consider how spina bifida may impact development and the key roles of the family, health care providers, and schools.

Chapter 2 is a review of the embryology and clinical features of neural tube defects. In Chapter 3, I review the epidemiology of spina bifida, also discussing genetic issues, folic acid, prevention, and screening programs. In 1996, the Food and Drug Administration issued their folic acid fortification mandate requiring all enriched flour, breads, rice, and pasta products to contain folic acid beginning in January 1998. The Centers for Disease Control and Prevention recently reported a 19 percent decline in the incidence of neural tube defects in the United States between January 1990 and December 1999, from 37.8 to 30.5 per 100,000 conceptions. This is an encouraging trend, but there remains much to do in educating the public about folic acid supplementation.

The subsequent chapters are arranged chronologically in the life of an individual with spina bifida. In addition to discussing medical and surgical issues, I present expected patterns of development and behavior in these chapters. Chapter 4 considers pregnancy and childbirth, and it includes advice about gathering information and seeking sources of health care. One remarkable new development is the advent of prenatal or fetal surgery. In 1994, doctors at Vanderbilt began trying various methods for closing spina bifida defects with the baby still in the mother's womb. Since then, many improvements have been made in the procedure, which is now being done in a few major medical centers. There are considerable risks involved, and it is not clear whether this treatment is better for the baby. The National Institute of Child Health and Human Development (NICHD) has funded the Management of Myelomeningocele Study (MOMS) to answer this question by means of a multicenter clinical trial (www.spinabifidamoms.com).

In Chapter 5 I focus on the newborn baby, dealing with closure and repair, shunting, and a number of medical issues that may arise. Chapter 6 is about infants and toddlers. Walking and bracing are stressed, as well as nutrition and toileting. In Chapter 7 I discuss preschoolers, and their pivotal issues of self-help skills and independence. Chapter 8 concerns the school-age child. Among a number of important health issues, I emphasize continence. Since 1997, the antegrade continence enema (ACE) procedure has become available in some treatment centers as a surgical solution to some children's problems with bowel incontinence. Chapter 8 also offers a detailed discussion of learning abilities and disabilities. Chapter 9 concerns the problems of spina bifida in adolescence and young adulthood. In addition to consideration of common medical problems affecting this age group, there is a discussion of sexuality, a vital area of concern that has been largely neglected in the medical community.

In Chapter 10 I examine family issues: the ways in which a child with spina bifida affects family functioning and the reciprocal effects of the family on the child. Also, I discuss financial matters and the impact of health care reform. I explore school issues in greater depth in Chapter 11 and also consider the world of work, which is of vital importance given the extremely low employment rates characteristically seen among adults with spina bifida. Of course, life is not only about work, and so I deal with the related issues of socialization and recreation.

Chapter 1 includes two personal accounts of the experience of spina bifida. The first is written by the parent of a child whom I have followed in our clinic. The second is written by an adult with spina bifida. I am very grateful to these two individuals for sharing their perspectives and giving me an opportunity to learn from them. In keeping with the spirit of the book, I have solicited the comments and advice of a number of parents of children with spina bifida regarding much of its content, and I have given these parents "the last word" at the end of most of the chapters in a section entitled "Parent-to-Parent." In letters I received from around the world since this book was first published, many parents who wrote to say that they found the book valuable specifically expressed their enjoyment of reading these pages. My sincere thanks to the Spina Bifida Association of America (www.sbaa.org) for their tireless advocacy and for providing me with an updated directory of resources, which appears in the Appendix. I am very grateful to all the people whose cumulative experience and wisdom I have organized on these pages.

Acknowledgments

Thanks to the following fine people for teaching, advising, and inspiring: Martin Bax, Maddie Blackburn, Todd Blumenthal, Nancy Cheschier, Pam Dixon, Walter Greene, Steve Gudeman, Holly Holland, John Holter, Cathy Howes, Pat Johnson, Ann Jones, Don Lollar, Michelle Macias, Joanne Mackey, Paula Mattocks, Susan McLaughlin, Jerry Oakes, Carol Sackett, Ben Skillman, Lynn Tuttle, and Gordon Worley. Thanks also to my illustrator, Pete Bedick, and my editors, Barbara Hanrahan and David Perry.

Glossary

Abduction	sideways movement of the limbs away from the midline
Adduction	sideways movement toward the midline
Alpha-fetoprotein (AFP)	a substance produced by a fetus that forms the basis of a screening test for spina bifida in pregnancy
Anencephaly	open neural tube defect with absent brain development, leading to early death
Anterior fontanel	the soft spot on the front of the head of an infant
Anticholinergic medication	drug used to relax the bladder
Apnea	period of absent breathing
Arthrodesis	the surgical fixation of a joint
Ataxia	a neurologic condition in which coordination of movement is impaired
Attention deficit	a specific difficulty with concentration that can impair school performance and social relationships
Autonomic nervous system	the nerves that regulate automatic functions of the body
Body cast	an immobilizing jacket that is molded to the legs and lower body
Brace	an aid for the support of a joint
Brainstem	the lower portion of the brain important for breathing and other vital functions
Calcaneovalgus	a foot deformity in which the heel is turned outward and the front part of the foot is elevated
Catheter	a hollow tube used to drain the bladder
Central nervous system	the brain and spinal cord
Cerebrospinal fluid (CSF)	the clear liquid that flows inside and outside the brain and spine

Cervical	pertaining to the neck
Chiari malformation	abnormal development of the lower part of the brain; frequently accompanies spina bifida
Clean intermittent catheterization (CIC)	a technique of inserting a catheter, draining a full bladder, and then removing the catheter
Clubfoot	foot deformity, usually talipes equinovarus
Coccyx	the tailbone of the spine
Cognitive	pertaining to functions of the brain such as thinking, learning, and processing information
Contractures	fixed deformities at the joints resulting in loss of range of motion
Corpus callosum	a midline structure in the brain
Cranium bifidum (encephalocele)	a defect in the skull with protrusion of brain tissue
Crede	a maneuver to empty the bladder by placing pressure on the lower abdomen
Cyanosis	dusky blue skin color usually due to severe breathing problems
Decubitus	an ulcer or sore on the skin as a result of pressure
Dermatomes	the areas of skin that get their sensation from different spinal nerves
Detrusor	the bladder muscle
Detrusor-sphincter dyssynergia (DSD)	failure of the bladder sphincter to open up when the bladder muscle contracts
Developmental delay	a significant lag between a child's age and his/her level of development (usually applies to children of three years or younger)
Disability	a lifelong condition affecting important activities or functions of daily living
Dislocated	a joint that is out of place, not in its socket
Dorsiflex	a backward bending of the forefoot at the ankle
Dura	the outer membrane of the meninges
Encephalocele	see cranium bifidum
Enema	a liquid medicine inserted into the rectum to stimulate a bowel movement
Equinovarus	similar to equinus, with additional inward turning of the forefoot

Equinus	deformity of the foot in which the heel is pulled up and the forefoot is pulled down
Eversion	movement of the foot in which the sole turns outward away from the midline
Expressive language	the ability to express ideas in words and sentences
Extension	the straightening of a joint; the opposite of flexion
Femur	the thighbone, extending from the pelvis to the knee
Flexion	the bending of a joint; the opposite of extension
Gait	the style of walking
Gastrocs	the calf muscles
Hamstrings	the large muscles at the back of the thigh
Handicap	an environmental or attitudinal barrier facing a person with a disability
Heel cord	the Achilles tendon below the calf muscle
Hip adductors	the muscles on the inside of the thigh that move the leg sideways toward the midline
Hydrocephalus	excessive cerebrospinal fluid in and around the brain
Hydronephrosis	widening and enlargement of the ureters and the collecting system of the kidneys
Hypertonia	a neurologic condition in which muscles have excessive contraction when they are stretched, that is, spasticity
Hypotonia	a neurologic condition of low tone, that is, floppiness
Ileal conduit	surgical procedure to drain the kidneys through an opening on the abdomen, thus bypassing the bladder
Impaction	severe constipation
Impairment	physical (or mental) problem in the individual that has the potential to interfere with functional activities
Incontinent	passing of urine or feces at unwanted or unexpected times
Inversion	movement of the foot in which the sole turns toward the midline
Kyphosis	a humplike curvature of the spine, commonly found in the region of the myelomeningocele
Learning disability	a specific difference in learning that leads to underachievement in school
Lipoma	swelling made of fat; sometimes found with myelomeningocele
Locomotion	moving by walking, crawling, or the like

Lordosis	an abnormally increased curvature of the spine, causing a hollow appearance in the lower back
Lumbar	the lower part of the back
Macrocephaly	an abnormally large head size
Meninges	fibrous sheaths that envelop the brain and spinal cord
Meningocele	a protrusion of the meninges, without brain or spinal cord, through a defect in the spine or skull
Mental retardation	below the normal range of cognitive ability
Microcephaly	an abnormally small head, usually accompanied by developmental delay
Myelomeningocele	a protrusion of spinal cord through a defect in the spine
Neural placode	abnormal, splayed-open nerve tissue at the site of the neural tube defect
Neural tube	the part of the embryo that develops into the brain and spinal cord
Neurogenic bladder	the condition of the bladder in spina bifida, in which it does not fill or empty normally
Neurosurgeon	a surgeon specializing in the treatment of brain and spinal cord problems
Occupational therapy	treatment based on the use of activities to help achieve maximum independence in daily-living skills
Orthopedic surgeon	a surgeon specializing in the treatment of bones, joints, and muscles
Orthosis	an appliance used to correct, prevent, or support deformities to improve function of movable body parts
Orthotist	a person specially trained in making and modifying orthoses to meet an individual's needs
Osteoporosis	brittle bones with deficient calcium; bones can fracture easily
Osteotomy	the surgical cutting of a bone to improve alignment
Paralysis	loss of muscle activity or movement
Paraplegia	paralysis of both legs
Parapodium	a crutchless standing device utilized for young children with paraplegia
Patella	the kneecap
Pediatrician	doctor who specializes in the treatment of children
Physiatrist	a physician who specializes in rehabilitation
Physical therapist	a health care professional who specializes in physical treatments to restore function and prevent disability

Plantar flexion	ankle flexed so that the foot is pointing upward
Prone	describing the position of a person lying horizontally on the abdomen, with the face turned downward
Proximal	closer to any point of reference
Pulmonary	pertaining to the lungs
Quadriceps	the group of muscles on the front of the thigh that extend the knee
Quadriplegia	paralysis of all four limbs
Rachischisis	a congenital condition in which the spinal cord is completely exposed and deformed
Range of motion	the full extent of movement of a particular joint
Receptive language	the ability to understand spoken language
Reciprocal	alternating, as feet alternate in walking
Reflex	an involuntary response to a specific stimulus
Reflux	abnormal backward flow of urine from the bladder up the ureters toward the kidneys
Reflux, gastro-esophageal	excessive regurgitation from the stomach into the esophagus
Related services	special services other than regular teaching that children may need to function effectively in school, for example, speech therapy, physical therapy, adaptive physical education (PE)
Renal	pertaining to the kidneys
Sacrum	the base of the spine that is firmly bound to the pelvis
Scoliosis	an abnormal sideways curvature of the spine
Shunt	a tube that connects two spaces, usually the ventricles with the peritoneal space in the abdomen
Soft tissue surgery	operations that involve lengthening muscles or tendons or releasing tight ligaments
Spasticity	permanently increased muscle tone
Sphincter	circular muscle surrounding an opening in the body
Spina bifida occulta	mild degree of neural tube defect covered completely with skin
Spinal fusion	an operation to make the spine stronger or more straight
Spinous processes	the bony projections at the back of the vertebrae
Standing frame	braces attached to a standing platform
Stoma	opening of the surgically diverted urinary conduit or bowel

Strabismus	squint or deviation of the eye
Stridor	a high-pitched or noisy breathing, especially when breathing in
Subluxation	a condition in which a joint begins to slip out of alignment
Supine	positioned lying horizontally on the back, with the face upward
Suppository	medicine, usually a softener or a stimulant laxative, inserted into the rectum
Swing-to gait	walking by putting both crutches forward and then lifting both feet and swinging them forward
Syrinx	a fluid-filled space in the spinal cord, usually in the neck, that can cause neurologic symptoms
Talipes equinovarus	typical clubfoot deformity, with heel inversion and foot plantar flexion
Talus	the bone of the foot that meets the tibia and fibula to form the main ankle joint
Tendon transfer	surgical procedure to move a tendon of a muscle so that the muscle pulls in another direction
Tenotomy	cutting a tendon to weaken its pull
Tethering	scarring around the spina bifida repair, so that the spine is pulled down abnormally low
Thoracic	pertaining to the chest or upper part of the trunk
Tibia	the larger bone in the lower leg, the shinbone
Tone	the degree of resistance of muscle to stretch
Two-point gait	walking by moving the right crutch and left leg together, then the left crutch and right leg
Ureters	tubes that carry urine from the kidneys to the bladder
Urethra	the tube through which urine naturally flows from the bladder during urination
Urodynamics	a detailed study of bladder pressures and urine flow
Urologist	a doctor who specializes in the treatment of urinary tract (kidneys, ureters, bladder, urethra) problems
Valgus	bent outward, away from the midline
Varus	bent inward, toward the midline
Ventricles	the interconnected spaces in the brain filled with cerebrospinal fluid
Ventriculitis	an infection of the ventricles, usually involving the shunt

Ventriculo-
   peritoneal
   shunt   plastic tube connecting the ventricles to the abdomen to treat hydrocephalus

Vertebrae   the bones of the spinal column (backbone)

Vestibular system   the inner ear and neurologic system that controls balance

Walker   movable aid used to provide stability in walking

Living with

Spina Bifida

CHAPTER 1

A Holistic Overview of Spina Bifida

A BRIEF CLINICAL DESCRIPTION

"Spina bifida" means a split or divided spine. It is a birth defect that occurs within the first month of pregnancy, when the embryo is about the length of a grain of rice. The cause of spina bifida is not known with certainty, but it is likely that folic acid deficiency during the crucial early weeks of pregnancy sometimes contributes to the problem.

The defect in the spine may occur anywhere along the spinal column but is usually found in the midback (thoracic), in the lower back (lumbar), or at the base of the spine (sacral). Spina bifida may be open or closed. Closed spina bifida, or "spina bifida occulta," is a fairly common condition in which the bones of the spine may be incomplete, but the defect is covered by skin and the spinal cord is usually normal. Most people with spina bifida occulta have no symptoms or clinical problems. Usually the term "spina bifida" is reserved for an open defect of the spine, in which the spinal cord does not form properly and is exposed (Figure 1.1). Another commonly used term for this condition is "myelomeningocele," in which there is generally some degree of paralysis of the muscles in the leg. If the defect is in the high-lumbar or thoracic region, there may be few functioning leg muscles, whereas lower defects may result in lesser degrees of paralysis. The nonfunctioning part of the spine may also cause loss of sensation in the legs and may give rise to orthopedic deformities. There is often some interference with normal bladder and bowel control. The clinical problems associated with spina bifida are described more fully in Chapter 2.

Most babies born with spina bifida also develop excess fluid in the ventricles (fluid spaces) in the brain. This problem is known as hydrocephalus and is typically treated in the newborn period with the placement of a shunt to drain the excess fluid. Hydrocephalus and its treatment are discussed in more depth in Chapter 5.

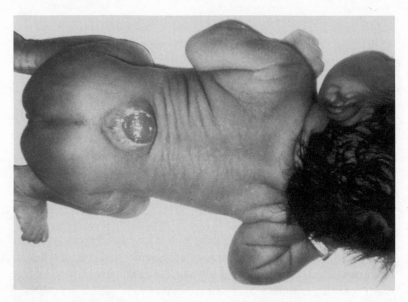

Figure 1.1. Spina bifida: a newborn infant with a midlumbar, open myelomeningocele

A DEVELOPMENTAL PERSPECTIVE

As I write this brief overview of spina bifida, I am working as camp doctor at a summer camp for children with this condition. Watching these youngsters playing and having fun, I see enormous variation in development. The outlook for the individual child is hard, if not impossible, to predict with any accuracy. A child's development unfolds in unique ways. Although our genetic makeup powerfully influences our development, environmental forces are equally critical. The destiny of the individual is therefore a product of both "nature" and "nurture" and the interplay between these two. A combination of good genes, a supportive family, and a facilitating environment can enable an individual to find ways around the physical limitations imposed by the presence of a birth defect.

Another important principle of development is that it does not occur smoothly but rather in fits and starts, with sudden growth periods and other quiet plateaus. Furthermore, the demands are continually changing. So it is that a child may have successfully met the demands and challenges of preschool and kindergarten but now begins to show learning problems in early elementary school. These problems do not truly arise out of the blue but were not evident in earlier years because the demands and expectations then were different from those now.

The key to maximizing developmental outcomes and fulfilling potential is to emphasize strengths and to build on them. Think "abilities," not disabilities, and focus on the strengths rather than the deficits. To put this principle into practice, professionals and families must work together as an effective partnership.

Studies that have followed large numbers of children with spina bifida into adulthood show many reasons to feel optimistic. For example, in Dr. D. G. McLone's study (McLone 1989), 85 to 90 percent of babies with spina bifida survived into adulthood, 70 to 80 percent had normal IQ scores, 80 percent were socially continent, and fully 75 percent were in competitive employment. These favorable statistics reflect advances in and a more aggressive, comprehensive approach toward treatment over the past fifteen years or so. Many adults with spina bifida did not have the benefit of such treatment approaches, however. This is reflected in the less favorable results of other follow-up studies. For example, Dr. Gillian Hunt (1990) published a study of young adults in the United Kingdom, showing a survival rate of 59 percent. Sixty-eight percent of her series had IQ scores of 80 or above, 52 percent were independent, 25 percent were continent, and only 25 percent were in competitive employment.

Promoting good health and optimal development is the most important challenge for people with spina bifida and their families. For all people with disabilities, prevention of further disability from secondary conditions is the key to meeting this challenge. Secondary conditions may include contractures of the joints, depression, obesity, and skin breakdown. Prevention of secondary conditions involves the elimination of risk factors for further deterioration; such prevention activities may depend on changing the individual's behavior, aspects of the environment, or both. This is the joint responsibility of the family and the health care providers. In this country and elsewhere, there is growing recognition of the critical importance of preventing secondary disability. Above all else, it is these activities that really make a difference over the life span of those with disabilities. The Disabilities Prevention Program of the Centers for Disease Control in Atlanta is especially interested in this issue, and the Americans with Disabilities Act (discussed in more depth in Chapter 11) has added additional impetus. These themes of health promotion, prevention of secondary disabilities, and the maximizing of developmental outcomes are stressed throughout this book. In later chapters we shall explore these themes as we consider spina bifida through the life span: how to promote good health, to prevent problems, and to improve quality of life at different ages. First, it is essential to define some important terms

---

Loss of sensation

Paralysis of muscle groups

Problems with bladder, bowel, and sexual function

Learning and developmental problems

Orthopedic problems

Figure 1.2. Impairments that commonly (but not always) occur in spina bifida

and discuss a framework for understanding disability. This framework is based on the World Health Organization's International Classification of Impairments, Disabilities, and Handicaps (1980).

IMPAIRMENTS, DISABILITIES, AND HANDICAPS

The main impairments of spina bifida are the sensory and motor impairments discussed above. In addition, there may be subtle cognitive impairments related to changes that occur in the developing baby's brain. These and other impairments of spina bifida are shown in Figure 1.2.

When an impairment significantly interferes with one or more major life activities of an individual, a disability can be said to exist. Not every impairment construes a disability. One can be extraordinarily tone-deaf and have a severe impairment in music appreciation, for example, yet one would hardly be described as music disabled! The key issue is the extent to which an impairment interferes with functional activities. The impact of an impairment on day-to-day function may be decreased by technology, equipment, and good ideas. Velcro has dramatically decreased the fine-motor disabilities of millions of people, for instance.

Disabilities are lifelong, although their relative importance and their impacts may change over time. A learning disability, for example, may be extremely evident in school, where academic demands are ever present, but an adult with a learning disability may choose an occupation that plays to his or her strengths, thus allowing progress and productivity. Choices, compromises, and adaptations enable an individual to live with a disability and rise above it.

"Handicap" is a term that is out of favor in this country. When a disability runs headlong into a barrier imposed by the environment, that is a handicap. Using a wheelchair is a handicap if there are no access ramps or if you can't use public transport. We cannot pretend that handicaps do not exist, but they exist largely in the realm of the environment, not in the person with a disability. By removing the barriers, be they physical or attitudinal, we remove the handicaps.

For individuals with spina bifida, a disability of locomotion is often the first to become evident. Spinal level and muscle strength are the most important determinants of a young child's readiness to walk. Toddlers with low-lumbar spina bifida may progress easily from reciprocal crawling to standing and may start to walk with only minimal bracing around the ankles. Those with higher lesions will need more extensive bracing to promote walking. Children are naturally motivated to be upright and ambulatory, and there are physical and psychological benefits to being up and walking, even if the bracing needs, gait training, and orthopedic procedures are extensive. For many children with midlumbar-level spina bifida or above, however, continued ambulation becomes impractical. Getting in and out of long leg braces can be time consuming, and the process of walking, extremely tiring. Many find a greater ease and efficiency in the use of wheelchairs, and as more and more places become wheelchair accessible, this option needs to be considered. Different kinds of braces and patterns of ambulation will be discussed in Chapter 6. The point here is that many youngsters may feel less disabled in a chair than in long leg braces.

Many young children with spina bifida and hydrocephalus have an impairment of fine-motor coordination. They may be less likely to explore toys with their hands and to manipulate objects with dexterity. Because the active exploration of the environment is an important precursor of learning in infancy, some of these children may be delayed in their acquisition of key visual-spatial concepts. It is not altogether surprising that many of these children struggle in mathematics and other aspects of learning in later years. I have also seen many children with spina bifida who lack the manual dexterity and eye-hand coordination to manage crucial challenges of self-care successfully, such as toileting and self-catheterization. In this way, a common impairment in spina bifida may give rise to a disability affecting learning and/or self-care. Generalized disability in learning and self-care is sometimes called "developmental disability."

The key to minimizing developmental disability is to maximize independence and self-care. Independence and self-care skills are acquired in sequence, in a step-by-step fashion. This is why it is so important to stimulate these fine-motor and adaptive skills early on. I strongly urge parents to encourage their infants to explore the world around them. It is important to overcome our natural parental tendencies to be overprotective of infants and toddlers with spina bifida, to let the little ones learn through doing, even if they have to work very hard in the process. It is through doing, through exploring, that we learn about cause and effect and develop our internal motivation. Early developmental intervention, involving parents and therapists, is the key to decreasing the developmental disability in spina bifida.

I have made an effort in this chapter to distinguish impairments, disabilities, and handicaps because these crucial distinctions need to be made for a child to fulfill his or her potential. Parents, teachers, and health care professionals alike must strive to remember that impairments need not necessarily become disabilities, and disabilities should never become handicaps.

At this point, I shall hand over the "pen" to people who really know what they are writing about! The first is an account of a young child, written by his mother. The second is an autobiographical note from an adult woman, who describes some of her firsthand experience of having spina bifida.

THE STORY OF A CHILD

My name is Kim. I am twenty-seven years old. My son Sam was born in May 1992 with spina bifida.

I first found out there was possibly a problem with my pregnancy at fifteen weeks when I had the AFP (alpha-fetoprotein) test done. This was my second child, and when they asked if I wanted the AFP test done, I still didn't know exactly what it was but remembered I had had it done when I was pregnant with my daughter. I remember my obstetrician telling me it had something to do with Down syndrome. So I decided I might as well have it done. I didn't give it much more thought. That is, until the day my obstetrician called me at work and told me my AFP had come back slightly elevated. "My what? Is what? What does that mean? Is my baby going to be all right?" My heart jumped to my throat, I could feel my pulse racing, I felt nauseous, and the tears started pouring. I had so many questions, and I was scared to death. I immediately made an appointment to have an ultrasound done in Chapel Hill. I then left work. I just had to!

Immediately, I began collecting information on the AFP test. By the next day I felt much better because I had read that only one or two out of every fifty women who have an initial high reading will have an affected fetus. This could never happen to me! On the day my husband Michael and I went to Chapel Hill for the ultrasound, I was a little nervous, but I just knew everything was going to be fine after all.

First, we had the counselor talk to us about spina bifida. She asked a few questions about our medical history. She helped us to understand what was going on and what to expect if the ultrasound did show a problem.

Now came time for the ultrasound. Almost immediately, the technician saw "something suspicious." Then the tears started flowing again. She went to get the doctor. Dr. Cheschier came in, looked at the ultrasound, and began explaining what she saw. I can't remember all that was said. I still couldn't believe this was happening to me.

After the ultrasound, Dr. Cheschier, Michael, and I went into her office and began discussing Sam's condition. The one good thing that came out of this day was that we found out that we were having a boy. From that day on the baby wasn't a fetus or an "it"; he was Sam.

The next step was to have an amniocentesis done. This was to make sure there were no other problems. The amnio confirmed spina bifida, but there were no other concerns.

Now the subject of terminating the pregnancy came up. Well, for me, I never had to think twice about it. I knew I wanted to keep Sam. Something deep inside of me kept telling me I was making the right decision. If the prognosis for Sam had been worse, if there had been other problems, I don't know that I would have made the same choice. I just knew that this was the right choice for me. As for my husband, who is Catholic, abortion was never even a possibility. And as for my family and friends, my decision to continue the pregnancy was questioned by them. I know in my heart their main concern was me. I remember several arguments with one of my best friends. She wanted to know what I was going to tell him when he asked why he couldn't run and play like all the other kids. How do you answer a question like that? I couldn't predict the future. I couldn't explain to people the calming feeling I had, knowing God would never put more on me than I could handle. This experience truly brought out my faith in God. I did a lot of praying.

For the next five months, my life revolved around doctor's appointments, gathering every bit of information I could find about spina bifida, working full time, spending every moment I could with my daughter, buying a house, keeping my sanity, being optimistic, and keeping a smile on my face. I had meetings with all the specialists. I remember meeting with Dr. Sandler, asking him a thousand questions, and wishing he had a crystal ball so he could answer them. Will Sam be able to walk, to play sports, to go to the bathroom, to have girlfriends, to go to college, to get married, to have a family? No one knew the answers.

As time went on, Sam's prognosis did seem to improve. The opening in Sam's spine was very low and small. I was told he could quite possibly have to use a wheelchair but that there was a good chance he would walk with leg braces. As far as the fluid developing in his head, I read that 90 percent of children develop hydrocephalus. We kept waiting for bad news, but Sam never developed it.

Then Sam was born May 6, 1992, at 10:00 A.M., in Chapel Hill. Sam weighed eight pounds, thirteen ounces, and was twenty inches long. He was beautiful!

Yes, he did have an opening in his spine, and he had to have surgery within the first few hours of his life. The operation went well. Sam was out of surgery in about three hours and went to the neonatal intensive care unit. I asked the doctors if Sam would be able to go home with me. Dr. Sandler said it was highly unlikely that a baby born with spina bifida would go home at the same time as the mother. Well, not only did Sam go home with me, he was in the ICU for only two days before he was moved to the regular nursery (although I kept him rooming in with me most of the time)!

Sam is now eighteen months old. He is walking, running, climbing, dancing, just like any other eighteen-month-old child. He did not develop hydrocephalus, and so he never had to have a shunt. Sam is unquestionably a miracle baby, and I know the chances of a child with spina bifida turning out to be this healthy are slim, but it happened. I don't regret any part of the experience I had. Some people think I would have been better off not knowing about the spina bifida, especially since he turned out to be so healthy. I don't agree. Because I was informed of the possibilities, I was able to give Sam the best care possible. I had the best doctors, the most advanced equipment, and was able to prepare myself mentally.

It was a miracle that Sam turned out the way he did, but if he had not I would have been ready. I can't begin to imagine what it would have been like if I had not known there were any problems until after he was born. I knew in advance that I would not be able to hold him immediately, and that was one of the hardest things to accept. However, I was able to prepare myself for that. Also, if I had not been informed of the situation in advance, as soon as Sam was born the doctors would have seen the hole, they would not have let me hold him, and I would have had no idea what was going on. Knowing how overwhelming that natural instinct is to want to hold your baby, well, I can't even begin to imagine the pain and terror I know I would have felt if I had not been prepared for Sam's birth.

If I had to go through this again, I would not change any decision I made. I believe in making informed choices, in having all the facts, and, most of all, in the power of prayer.

AN ADULT'S STORY

Being a person with spina bifida has meant many things to me. Having spina bifida has meant that I have to work twice as hard at things that come naturally to some people, such as trying to walk, to take care of myself, and to make my own living. These things have been hard at times, but not nearly as difficult as trying to get other people to see me as "normal" and treat me as they would anyone else. Most people are very nice when they meet me, but a lot of them seem to think that I'm someone to pity or treat differently than they would someone who can walk normally. For me, that's been the most difficult thing about spina bifida, being treated as if I'm different just because I walk on crutches. As a child, it was hard to go out in public and be stared at by people and pointed at and talked about by kids, but I learned to just go on as if I didn't hear or see them, because I knew the kids didn't know any better, and neither did the adults if they had never been around someone with a disability. I learned to ignore all that, but it didn't make it any easier. I think that having to face situations like that has made me stronger and more determined to prove to everyone that I am normal and as capable of taking care of myself as anyone else.

Luckily, I've had very supportive family and friends. My parents have always encouraged and always told me that there was nothing I couldn't do if I wanted to badly enough. God has given me a lot of strength and determination also, which has helped me through some very difficult times.

Even though my parents have been very supportive of my wanting to become independent, they have been supportive only to a point. They wanted me to be independent, but not too independent! They kind of wanted to define what they thought independent should mean for me. They wanted me to go to college and get a degree and a job, but they didn't like it when I started driving and going places without them and making my own decisions without consulting them first. It's been hard for my parents to let go, but I think I've proven to them that I can take care of myself and that I will be just fine.

Having spina bifida has meant that I have had to try twice as hard as other people to become independent, but it has made me a much stronger person because of it. And what's more, I don't take my independence and my accomplishments for granted. Living on my own, making my own living, and coming and going as I please means more to me than I can say, and I know that I have worked hard to achieve all this. I believe my disability and the obstacles I've had to overcome because of it have made me stronger, and they have made me who I am. So in a way, my disability has been an advantage. It has made me strong enough to handle situations and disappointments that I might not have been strong enough to handle otherwise.

Neural Tube Defects

W hat are neural tube defects? How do they arise in the human embryo? What are the clinical features of spina bifida, and how do these changes in the embryo give rise to later problems in the child with spina bifida? Answers to these questions are essential for parents and professionals who want fully to understand this condition. In this chapter, I will begin by reviewing what is known about *how* the complex birth defect of spina bifida occurs. (As much as we know about *why* it occurs will be presented in the section on epidemiology in Chapter 3.) Next, because not all spina bifida birth defects look the same, I will describe the different forms of spina bifida. Finally, I will present the functional problems associated with spina bifida and explain how they are related to the underlying birth defect.

THE EMBRYOLOGY OF NEURAL TUBE DEFECTS

To understand more completely the nature of neural tube defects, this chapter begins with the first part of the miraculous development of the human embryo. A single cell, the fertilized egg, rapidly divides and divides again to form a sphere, which begins to differentiate into a tiny disk from which the embryo itself develops. The disk, barely a millimeter in length, or the size of a comma, includes an inner layer (endoderm), which will give rise to the gut; a middle layer (mesoderm), from which will develop the heart and circulatory system, muscles, and bones; and an outer layer (ectoderm), from which the skin and central nervous system develop.

We pick up events at around eighteen days (Figure 2.1). The part of the ectoderm that is to become the nervous system (the neurectoderm) is made up of two neural folds running from the head to the tail of the embryo, which still measures less than two millimeters (the length of a sesame seed). As the crests of the neural folds rise like waves on the surface

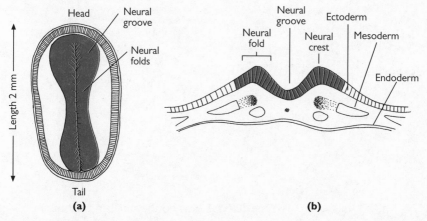

Figure 2.1. The human embryo at eighteen days, showing the view from above (a) and a cross-sectional view (b). Notice how the two neural folds are in the process of coming together to form a tube covered by skin.

of the embryo, pulling the primitive skin with them, they gradually move closer together and unite in the midline. In this way, the neural tube begins to form, with the skin providing a continuous covering above it. It usually does so in the region of the embryo that will later become the cervical and upper-thoracic spinal cord. In the following few days, the tube extends in both directions as the neural crests come together. By thirty days, the embryo measures three to five millimeters (the size of a grain of rice), and the neural tube has been formed along its length, with openings at either end (the anterior and posterior neuropores). It is the failure of this crucial process of neural tube formation (neurulation) that underlies open spina bifida (Figure 2.2).

The open neural tube is only part of the overall picture of abnormal development of the central nervous system seen in spina bifida. Almost all children with spina bifida also have a complex brain malformation known as the Arnold-Chiari II malformation. This will be discussed in greater depth in Chapter 5. The Chiari malformation consists of the downward displacement of the cerebellum, the elongation and downward displacement of the medulla and fourth ventricle, a small posterior fossa, and accompanying hydrocephalus.

One of the questions that has puzzled neuroscientists is the link between the open neural tube and these other abnormalities. It has long been argued that these other changes occurred much later in fetal life by the downward traction of the spinal cord on the brain. The abnormal spinal cord is

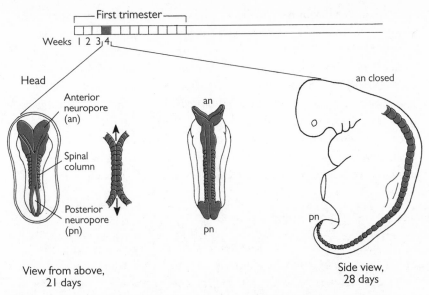

Figure 2.2. The formation of the neural tube. In just seven days, the tube has closed like a two-directional zipper. At this time, the embryo is the size of a grain of rice.

usually tethered to surrounding tissues, and it was thought that this tended to pull the brainstem down. In their work with the Splotch mouse animal model, Drs. McLone and Knepper (1989) found convincing evidence that the Chiari malformation occurs much earlier in the development of the embryo. Previous research (Desmond 1982) demonstrated that the neural tube of normal human embryos becomes blocked for forty-eight to seventy-two hours, while glycoproteins are laid down on the inner walls of the tube. Scanning electron micrographs of normal Splotch mice show the same process occurring around the eleventh day (equivalent to day thirty-five in the human embryo). In Splotch mice with neural tube defects, however, this occlusion of the tube did not occur, and there was evidence that the glycoproteins were not being synthesized and laid down. The significance of all this is that the transient blockage leads to an accumulation of fluid and pressure in the developing brain vesicles. These outpouchings of neural tissue become progressively distended, causing the posterior fossa to develop its usual size and shape. If the neural tube remains open, the dynamic fluid and pressure changes in the primitive ventricular system do not occur, and as a result, the posterior fossa remains small. No longer is it able to accommodate the developing hindbrain, which has no alternative but to herniate upward through a malformed, low-lying tentorium and downward, through a large foramen magnum. Moreover, a number of other subtle abnormalities of Chiari malformation become evident. The corpus callosum does not form properly, and the massa intermedia is enlarged as a result of the disturbed sequence of development. Even the formation of the overlying skull bone is affected, so that the collagen bundles are disorganized, and the bone has a characteristic appearance (*luckenschadel*). Lastly, the circulation of cerebrospinal fluid is frequently affected by obstruction at the aqueduct, at the outlets of the fourth ventricle, or both. This leads to the development of hydrocephalus, which is often progressive, later in the life of the fetus.

THE ANATOMY OF SPINA BIFIDA

When the normal closure of the neural tube is disrupted or disturbed, there is a range of anatomic abnormalities that may ensue. Some newborns may have large lesions containing the splayed-open, abnormal nerve tissue of the spine (the neural placode), whereas others may have little evidence of the underlying malformation of the spine.

Spina Bifida Occulta

When the underlying neural tube defect is completely covered with skin, the condition is known as spina bifida occulta—that is, hidden spina bifida. Frequently, there are telltale signs on close examination of the back. There may be a defect in the vertebrae or spine bones, or the skin overlying the defect may be dimpled, thickened, pigmented, or hairy. In some cases, there is a soft swelling overlying the spine, composed of fatty tissue (lipoma). These may be simple lipomas, unassociated with neural tube defects, but more often there are associated neural tube defects, in which case they are known as lipomeningoceles. Not infrequently, the fatty tissue extends into the spinal canal, where it can expand and press on the spinal cord. Although there may be no motor or sensory impairments evident at birth, subtle, progressive neurologic deterioration often becomes evident in later childhood or adulthood. Foot deformities, scoliosis, pain, or weakness may herald the progression of these problems. Most neurosurgeons advocate for early and aggressive surgical removal of intraspinal lipomas before these troublesome and usually irreversible symptoms occur.

In many instances, however, spina bifida occulta is so mild that there is no disturbance of spinal function at all. The arches of the vertebrae may be incomplete, but the spinal cord itself is normal, there is no lipoma,

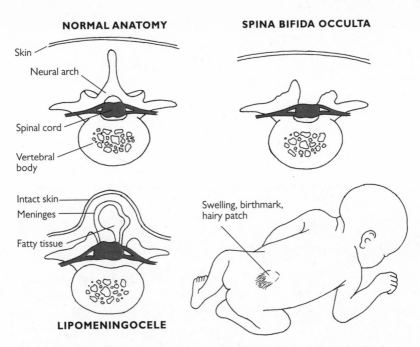

NORMAL ANATOMY

Skin
Neural arch
Spinal cord
Vertebral body

Intact skin
Meninges
Fatty tissue

LIPOMENINGOCELE

SPINA BIFIDA OCCULTA

Swelling, birthmark, hairy patch

Figure 2.3. The spectrum of spina bifida occulta. Abnormalities of this kind are common (occurring in 3–5 percent of the population) and usually do not cause any problems.

and there are no neurologic abnormalities evident. Spina bifida occulta of this sort probably occurs in 3–5 percent of the population and is usually a chance finding that is of no clinical significance. In fact, it is not uncommon that a parent of a baby with spina bifida confides in the doctor that he or she has a hairy patch but has never had any symptoms to suggest spinal cord problems (Figure 2.3).

Spina bifida occulta may be easily confirmed with X-rays. However, if there are abnormal neurologic signs, pain, numbness, or changes in posture, gait, or bladder function, a magnetic resonance imaging (MRI) scan is usually the best method of visualizing associated spinal cord problems.

Open Spina Bifida

Open spina bifida occurs when the neural tube defect is not covered over with skin (Figure 2.4). Without a skin covering, it is the nerve tissue itself that is present at the surface of the baby's back. Usually there is the splayed-open, malformed spinal cord (neural placode), as well as the fibrous sheath (meninges) that typically surrounds the spinal cord. Hence,

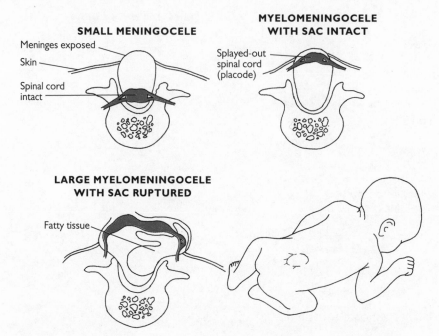

Figure 2.4. Myelomeningoceles and the spectrum of open spina bifida. Neural elements, including the splayed-out spinal cord, the meninges, and fatty tissue may all be exposed at the surface of the baby's back.

this appearance is known as myelomeningocele or meningomyelocele (where "myelo" means "spine" and "cele" means "swelling"). Very small lesions, usually in the sacrum (the lower part of the spine) that do not appear to contain spinal cord are called meningoceles. Excessive fatty tissue is sometimes present as well (lipomyelomeningocele). The myelomeningocele is often saclike, with an intact layer of meninges surrounding a collection of cerebrospinal fluid (CSF). In many cases, the fragile sac is disrupted, perhaps during delivery, so that CSF leaks from the myelomeningocele.

Myelomeningoceles are quite variable in size and location. Some may be confined to one or two vertebral levels, and the placode may measure only two or three centimeters in length. Others may be far more extensive, extending ten or more centimeters along the vertebral column. The functional impact of a myelomeningocele depends much more on its uppermost level than on its size, as I shall discuss in the next section. In other words, a small lesion at the level of the first lumbar vertebra (L1) is likely to lead to a disturbance of function similar to that caused by a large lesion extending all the way from the fifth lumbar vertebra up to the first. Large lesions may present special problems of closure to the surgeon and may be accompanied by less stability of the spine and greater risk of scoliosis, but it is the level *below which the spinal cord does not work properly* that is of the greatest importance with respect to walking.

Anencephaly

Anencephaly, like spina bifida, is a neural tube defect. It arises from a failure in closure of the primitive neural tube and shares many of the known risk factors. The two conditions can frequently be caused in animals by the same experimental conditions in the laboratory. In anencephaly, the skull does not form, and the entire brain above the brainstem fails to develop. Unlike spina bifida, the condition is completely inoperable and the prognosis uniformly grim for those who are not stillborn. There is no capacity for learning or development, and inevitably, affected babies die, usually from failure to breathe or from infection. Ethical issues surrounding the use of anencephalic babies' organs for transplantation have arisen in recent years but are beyond the scope of this book.

Cranium Bifidum (Encephalocele)

For completeness, I will mention the related condition of cranium bifidum, more commonly known as encephalocele. This too develops early in pregnancy, possibly as a result of the neural tube failing to separate from the surrounding surface ectoderm in the embryo's developing head. It is usually associated with Chiari II malformations and may occur in conjunction with spina bifida. Encephaloceles, which are in essence protrusions of brain and meninges through a defect in the skull, are usually found in the midline at the back of the head (75 percent), and, less commonly, in the parietal area (15 percent), frontal skull, or upper part of the face. In the Far East, frontal encephaloceles are more common. They may be small and cystic (cranial meningoceles), in which case the prognosis following closure is excellent. Sometimes, however, they can contain a large volume of brain tissue, so that the rest of the brain is small, poorly developed, and severely hydrocephalic (Figure 2.5).

NEUROLOGIC IMPAIRMENTS IN SPINA BIFIDA

The complex clinical issues in spina bifida can be better understood by considering how the anatomy of spina bifida relates to the physical impairments that are commonly seen. I will first describe the primary neurologic

**OCCIPITAL
MENINGOCELE**

**SEVERE ENCEPHALOCELE
WITH HYDROCEPHALUS**

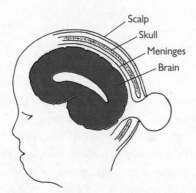
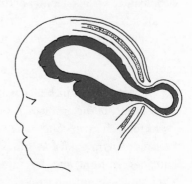

Figure 2.5. Encephaloceles: protrusions of brain and meninges through a defect in the skull

impairments that occur as a result of spina bifida and then the secondary impairments, or the way in which the primary neurologic impairments can affect other parts of the body and disturb other bodily functions.

Primary Impairments

Sensory Impairments

Throughout its length, the spinal cord contains nerve cells that receive information from the skin, joints, and muscles (Figure 2.6). These sensory nerves make connections in the spinal cord, thereby transmitting signals to the brain.

Sensations of touch, pressure, temperature, pain, and body position are in this way dependent on intact function of sensory nerves. The different levels of the spinal cord are responsible for receiving and transmitting sensations from different parts of the body: the sensory nerves in the lower cervical cord get sensation from the neck and shoulders; the lower thoracic nerves, from the abdominal area around the level of the umbilicus; and the lower lumbar nerves, from the side of the legs and the top of the feet, for example. These sensory "dermatomes" are shown in Figure 2.7. At the site where the neural tube fails to close, the sensory nerves do not form properly; thus sensation is impaired or absent. Moreover, sensations from below the neural tube defect are also absent because they cannot be transmitted up through the abnormally developed section of the spine. Therefore almost all individuals with myelomeningocele have a "sensory level" that can be determined on neurologic examination. I say "almost all" be-

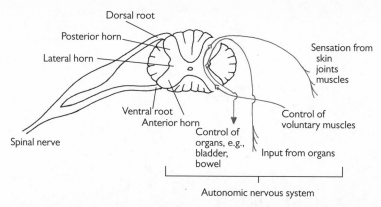

Dorsal root

Posterior horn

Lateral horn

Sensation from
skin
joints
muscles

Ventral root
Anterior horn

Spinal nerve

Control of
voluntary muscles

Control of
organs, e.g.,
bladder,
bowel

Input from organs

Autonomic nervous system

Figure 2.6. The structure and function of the spinal cord shown in cross section. Sensory nerves enter the dorsal root of the spinal cord, and the nerves that control voluntary muscles and the organs (such as the bladder and bowel) exit from the ventral root.

cause occasionally, partial sensation is preserved. Individuals with lower sacral lesions may have no detectable sensory loss. The loss of sensation has important implications, as we shall see in subsequent chapters. Just recently, for example, I saw an infant in clinic who was teething and had taken to chewing on his toes. Unfortunately, the lack of sensation caused him to chew large ulcers on his feet! Burns are another important hazard, against which parents must take special precautions. It is also worth noting that sensory levels may be asymmetrical, somewhat higher on one side than on the other. Interestingly, some people with spina bifida have reported that they have spontaneously developed small areas of sensation in areas that were previously completely numb. It would indeed be a dramatic breakthrough to learn ways of stimulating sensation in spina bifida. Unfortunately, most cases of changing sensation are losses of sensation, representing tethering of the spinal cord or some other complication of spina bifida.

Motor Impairments

Just as the sensory nerves at the level of the neural tube defect do not develop normal function, so too are the motor nerves affected (see Figure 2.8). Different muscle groups are supplied by nerves from different spinal levels. Hip flexors are controlled by nerves from the upper lumbar spine (L1); knee extensors, by midlumbar nerves; and so on. The figure shows the names of muscles important for walking and their corresponding nerve supply. A myelomeningocele at the low thoracic region (let's

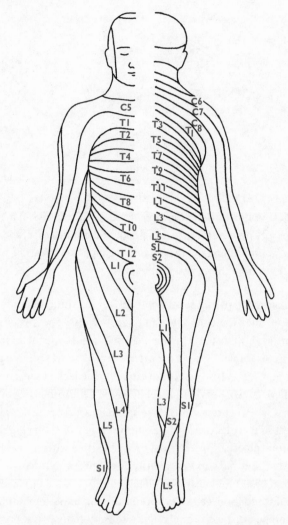

Figure 2.7. Dermatomes: the strips of skin for which sensation is supplied by the various levels of the spinal cord

say T12) may be expected to interfere with hip flexion, although some of the muscle fibers may be supplied by nerves from just above the lesion, leaving the individual with partial strength. You will recall that the sensory impairment of spina bifida extends below the lesion. In a similar way, the disruption of normal spine development in spina bifida interrupts the connections from the brain to motor nerves below the meningomyelocele. Thus, we would expect that a person with T12 spina bifida would have no controllable muscle function in other muscle groups in the legs. Nonvolitional or reflexic movement can sometimes be observed, espe-

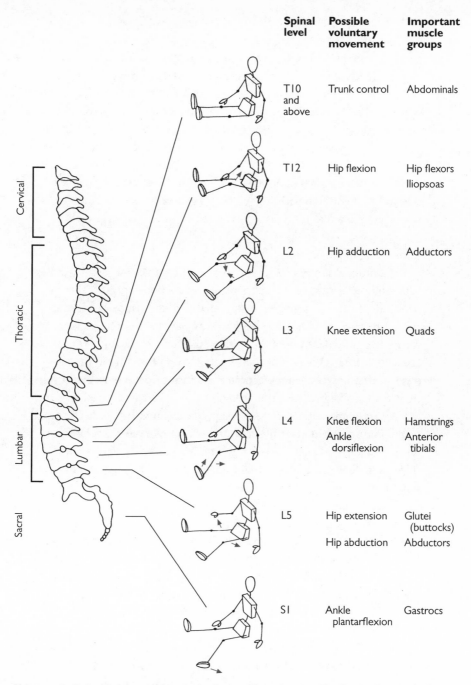

Spinal level	Possible voluntary movement	Important muscle groups
T10 and above	Trunk control	Abdominals
T12	Hip flexion	Hip flexors Iliopsoas
L2	Hip adduction	Adductors
L3	Knee extension	Quads
L4	Knee flexion Ankle dorsiflexion	Hamstrings Anterior tibials
L5	Hip extension Hip abduction	Glutei (buttocks) Abductors
S1	Ankle plantarflexion	Gastrocs

Figure 2.8. Spinal levels and the range of motor impairment. The figure shows which important muscle groups are likely to remain functional with different spinal levels.

cially in newborns, but this kind of movement is not under the control of the individual and does not have significance for later walking. The term paraplegia simply refers to absent muscle function in the legs. There are different levels of paraplegia in spina bifida, and these are generally classified as thoracic, high-lumbar (L1 or L2), midlumbar (L3), low-lumbar (L4 or L5), and sacral (S1). This primary motor impairment may result in secondary orthopedic impairments and disability of locomotion. The significance of these levels for subsequent bracing needs and walking abilities will be discussed in Chapter 6. Suffice it to say here that the prognosis for walking is excellent for all but thoracic and high-lumbar myelomeningocele and that children with higher lesions generally require more extensive bracing to walk.

Autonomic Impairments

In addition to motor and sensory nerves, the spinal cord also gives rise to autonomic nerves that help to control the function of organs. There are two kinds of autonomic nerves: parasympathetic and sympathetic. Of special importance in spina bifida are the sacral parasympathetic nerves that supply the muscular walls of the bladder, urethra, and rectum. Arising in the lowest or sacral region of the spinal cord and traveling to the pelvic organs, these nerves are important in the transmission of sensations from these organs—for example, the sensation of a full bladder or full rectum. Sacral parasympathetic nerves also supply the smooth muscle of these organs and are essential for the coordinated contractions that must occur for the bladder and rectum to empty completely. The sympathetic nerves that originate in the lumbar spinal cord play a role as well, controlling the important sphincters at the bladder outlet.

The autonomic nerves, especially the parasympathetic system, are also important in sexual functions. Stimulation of these nerves in sexual arousal causes the blood vessels supplying the sexual organs to dilate, leading to erection of the penis or the clitoris and lubrication of the vagina. Orgasm is accompanied by rhythmic contractions of smooth muscle under parasympathetic control. In the male, sympathetic contraction of the bladder sphincter also occurs, thereby preventing so-called retrograde ejaculation into the bladder.

Almost all individuals with spina bifida have bladder and bowel dysfunction, and most, but by no means all, adults with spina bifida have varying degrees of sexual dysfunction as a result of autonomic nerve impairment. Bladder, bowel, and sexual dysfunction are described in the section below on secondary impairments.

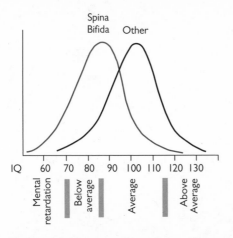

Areas of relative strength

Social cognition
Phonological processing
Long-term memory
Expressive language
Reading
Spelling

Common areas of weakness

Attention/organizational deficits
Impaired abstract reasoning
Visual-perceptual impairments
Poor eye-hand coordination
Poor visual-motor integration
Writing
Mathematics

Figure 2.9. Neurocognitive characteristics of spina bifida: typical patterns of performance. The figure shows the wide range of IQ scores among children with spina bifida, along with typical areas of strength and weakness.

Cognitive Impairments

Spina bifida is not just a condition of the spine. As discussed earlier in this chapter, there are associated abnormalities of the brain, most notably hydrocephalus and the Chiari malformation, in the majority of affected individuals. It is therefore logical to consider the effects on the brain as primary impairments of spina bifida. Not every individual with spina bifida has discernible cognitive impairments, and of those who do, the problems are often quite subtle. Nevertheless, they are sufficiently common, and the patterns of dysfunction are fairly characteristic. Figure 2.9 shows the features that characterize the cognitive impairments of spina bifida.

Individuals with spina bifida frequently have below average cognitive ability, and mild degrees of mental retardation are not uncommon. Abstract reasoning and visual-perceptual abilities are often the most impaired areas. Eye-hand coordination may be relatively poor, and reaction times, slow. Sequencing and organizational skills may be impaired. Although these difficulties are most often seen in children who have hydrocephalus, this is not always the case. There are some children with spina bifida but no hydrocephalus who have evidence of these impairments. It is not surprising that cognitive impairment can have an impact on the acquisition of academic skills, thereby constituting a learning disability, which will be discussed in Chapter 8.

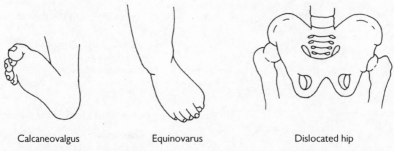

Calcaneovalgus   Equinovarus   Dislocated hip

Figure 2.10. Common orthopedic impairments in spina bifida: two forms of clubfoot and a dislocated hip

Secondary Impairments

Orthopedic Impairments

Muscles work in pairs around a joint: to move a joint, one group of muscles must contract, while the opposing group of muscles must relax. This fine balance between opposing muscle groups is key to coordinated movement and stability around a joint. Special problems can occur in spina bifida when the two groups are supplied by nerves from different spinal segments. Hip flexors, for example, are supplied by L1–L2 nerves, whereas hip extensors are supplied by L4–L5 nerves. If the spina bifida affects the lower lumbar spine, such that the hip extensors are not functional and the flexors are strong and unopposed, the resulting imbalance can lead to dislocation or partial dislocation (subluxation) of the hip joint. In some circumstances, the joints can become tight or contracted, problems that can profoundly affect the efficiency of locomotion. Contractures at the hips, knees, or ankles can greatly increase the energy needed for ambulation (Figure 2.10).

The most common orthopedic impairment evident at birth in babies with spina bifida is clubfoot. This impairment usually results from imbalance between muscle groups acting on the foot or because the paralysis of the legs in utero prevented sufficient movement of the fetus such that the foot was in effect caught in an unusual position. Another important orthopedic impairment that is secondary to muscle imbalance is scoliosis. As we shall see in Chapter 8, this can become a major problem later in childhood, especially in those with thoracic spina bifida.

Bladder Dysfunction

Urination begins with the sensation of bladder fullness and the urge to urinate. The process depends on the coordinated contraction of the

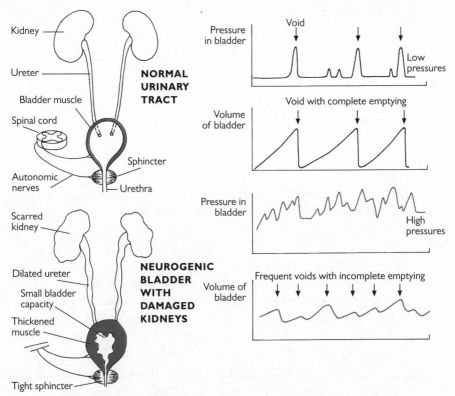

Figure 2.11. The mechanism of bladder dysfunction in spina bifida. In the normal urinary tract, pressures in the bladder remain low during filling, and the bladder is relaxed between voids. In the neurogenic bladder, there are often high pressures, a nonrelaxing bladder, and frequent voids with incomplete emptying, which can lead to kidney damage.

smooth muscle of the bladder (the detrusor muscle) and the simultaneous relaxation of the sphincters at the bladder outlet. Children with myelo-meningocele have impaired autonomic function and may therefore have absent or minimal sensation of bladder fullness and an inability to initiate the voluntary, coordinated process of urination. The so-called neurogenic bladder, freed from the inhibitory action of higher centers in the brain, does not relax sufficiently and therefore has a limited capacity. Further-more, the bladder sphincters may fail to open, with contraction of the bladder smooth muscle possibly leading to dramatic and sometimes dan-gerous increases in pressure. This "detrusor-sphincter dyssynergia" may cause distension of the ureters and kidneys (hydronephrosis) and kidney damage (Figure 2.11).

Bowel Dysfunction

A comparable disruption of the process of bowel emptying occurs, such that there may be no sensation of fullness in the rectum and little or no control over the release of stool. Because of the neurogenic bowel, stool tends to build up in the rectum and the distal colon, becoming harder and more difficult to pass. As the stool accumulates, the bowel walls are stretched and thinned, which further interferes with bowel function and aggravates the constipation. Moreover, as I shall describe in Chapter 6, constipation can interfere with bladder function and predispose one to urinary tract infections. Thus close attention needs to be paid to infants and toddlers with bowel dysfunction early on in order to optimize bowel management and achieve continence in later years.

Sexual Dysfunction

At the outset of any discussion of sexuality, it is very important to recognize that being a sexual being goes way beyond the discussion of sexual function—the purely biological considerations of the sexual organs and how they work. Sexuality involves love, intimacy, and the giving and receiving of pleasure. It resides in a vast domain of mind-body and human relationships, rather than in the mundane one of physiology and plumbing! I shall discuss some aspects of sexuality in greater depth in Chapter 9 on adolescents and young adults. Issues of sexuality and sexual expression are of vital concern to individuals with spina bifida and to parents of affected children. It is an area that the medical community has sadly neglected, perhaps out of a sense that this subject was "off limits." Very little research has been done, even concerning the basic descriptive, biological information about sexual function and dysfunction among individuals with spina bifida. Certainly, many individuals with spina bifida do have to deal with a variety of sexual dysfunctions related to autonomic nerve impairments. There appears to be considerable variation in the nature and extent of these dysfunctions, however, and it is not at all clear what accounts for this variation. It is also true that the majority of adults with spina bifida have pleasurable sexual sensations, and some have orgasms. Some men are able to maintain erections and even ejaculate (Sandler et al. 1995). The point is that the sexual dysfunctions of spina bifida should not greatly curtail the avenues for sexual fulfillment or in any way negate individuals' sexual beings.

Epidemiology of Spina Bifida

S pina bifida is, to a very large extent, a preventable condition. This statement may come as a surprise to some, but then in previous decades it would have been equally shocking to hear that phenylketonuria (PKU) and congenital hypothyroidism were preventable. Progress in the prevention of these two diseases rested heavily on the science of epidemiology, the study of the patterns of diseases in populations. In this chapter, I will discuss the epidemiology of spina bifida and explain my somewhat controversial position regarding its preventability. After presenting the evidence that suggests a nutritional cause of spina bifida, I also speculate about other possible genetic and environmental causes and consider approaches to the prevention of spina bifida. Prenatal screening programs and the use of such technologies as alpha-fetoprotein testing and ultrasound will be discussed. The chapter ends with a projection of possible prenatal medical and surgical treatments that may be on the horizon, including in utero surgery.

THE INCIDENCE OF SPINA BIFIDA

Studying the incidence of a condition in different geographic regions, among ethnic groups, or in the same population over time is like reading a good mystery novel! Therein lie the clues to a deeper understanding of the causes and associations of a disease. Of course, incidence rates are highly dependent on accurate record keeping. Although some countries have a long history of maintaining careful registers of birth defects, this practice is by no means widespread, so it is not always easy to obtain good and reliable data or to compare figures that were generated in different places and by different methods. In addition to these ascertainment problems, we also run into problems when we try to make comparisons based on birth records compiled since the advent of prenatal diagnosis and elective abortion of affected fetuses. Even if there were no change in the incidence of affected fetuses, the number of babies born with spina bifida would have decreased because of prenatal diagnosis. The *apparent* decline in incidence of spina bifida in the United States over the past ten years far exceeds the *real* decline for this reason. In spite of these difficulties, there is much to learn from the variations in incidence in different places, different times, different people, and different living conditions.

Comparisons between different countries are the most difficult to interpret, yet are striking in their disparity. The incidence in China is 100–200 per 10,000, whereas it is only 5–10 per 10,000 in the United States. To put this into perspective, three thousand babies with spina bifida are born each year in the United States and about one hundred thousand in China! What accounts for this enormous difference? The short answer, of course, is that we don't know. It is very difficult to tease apart the separate contributions of genes and environment, of "nature" and "nurture."

It is perhaps more fruitful to examine regional variations within a country. For example, there is an unusually high incidence in Northern Ireland and Wales compared with the rest of the United Kingdom. In the United States the mountainous country extending from New England down to Georgia, known as Appalachia, has a similarly high incidence. This regional influence seems to be environmental, because populations that move to these areas seem to have incidence rates similar to those of more indigenous populations, whereas groups that move to other areas have lower incidence rates. If specific environmental influences accounting for these regional variations could be found, this would have enormous implications for prevention. To date, unfortunately, no such factors have been identified. Examination of trends in incidence over time, however, can be revealing (Figure 3.1).

Evidence indicates, for example, that there was an epidemic of spina bifida in the United Kingdom in the 1870s and one in the United States in the 1930s. From 1970 to 1976, before the advent of prenatal diagnosis, the incidence in the United States fell from eight to four per ten thousand. Previous epidemics and these more recent changes in incidence in stable populations are not consistent with a predominantly genetic cause of spina bifida, for the incidence of genetic conditions, such as cystic fibrosis, stays quite constant over time if the gene pool remains stable. The changes in incidence of spina bifida over time are entirely consistent with environmental causes. Periods of high incidence correspond to times of poverty and social upheaval, the most notable being the Great Depression. This certainly suggests the possibility of important nutritional fac-

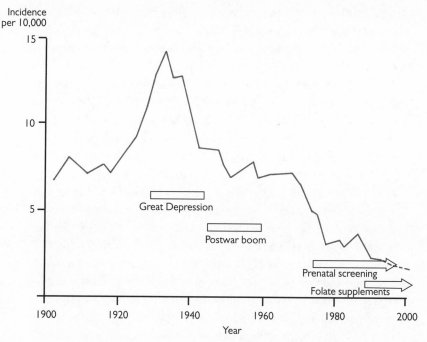

Figure 3.1. Approximate incidence of spina bifida in the United States since 1900. Note the peak during the years of the Great Depression. The decrease in the 1970s to fewer than five per ten thousand began before the widespread use of prenatal screening programs.

tors. Furthermore, when one examines the incidence within a population at a given time, one finds a significant socioeconomic gradient, such that poorer people have a higher incidence of spina bifida.

Folic Acid and the Role of Nutritional Deficiencies

A study in Yorkshire, England, and a similar one in the United States involving interviews and careful food records showed significant differences in the daily intake of a variety of nutrients between pregnant women of different social classes. If their diets are different, is it possible that a nutritional deficiency early in pregnancy explains the social class gradient in incidence rates?

In one study in Wales, pregnant women who had already had a previous baby with spina bifida were grouped into those who had "good diets" and those with "poor diets." There were no second spina bifida babies born to mothers in the former group, whereas 13 of 362 pregnancies in the latter group resulted in babies with spina bifida. This is a compelling difference but tells us nothing about which specific nutrients might be important.

A study in Western Australia used detailed twenty-four-hour food records to compare the dietary intake of specific nutrients among women who had given birth to a baby with spina bifida, those who had given birth to babies with other congenital problems, and those with normal babies. It was found that the risk of having a baby with spina bifida increased with lower intake of dietary folic acid.

In the United States, the use of nonprescription multivitamin preparations is common. Most of these contain folic acid in addition to vitamins. Mulinare et al. (1988) reported a study in which 347 mothers of babies with spina bifida were interviewed, as well as 2,829 control mothers. It was found that mothers of babies with spina bifida consumed a significantly lower number of vitamins. In this kind of study, however, there is no way of knowing with certainty whether it is the multivitamin consumption itself or some other health behavior that may be associated with vitamin use that is responsible. Maybe the women who took vitamins did not smoke or drink alcohol. Another problem with evidence of this sort is recall bias, that is, the tendency to try to explain the birth of a baby with a birth defect by racking our brains to think of possible reasons. Such retrospective data are likely to overestimate risk factors and are not as strong as prospective data.

Milunsky et al. (1989) prospectively interviewed 22,715 women who were undergoing amniocentesis about their use of multivitamins. Forty-nine of these women were subsequently found to have fetuses with neural tube defects. Neural tube defects were three times more likely among those women who were not taking vitamins or who took vitamins after the sixth week of pregnancy than among those who took folic acid during the first six weeks (Figure 3.2). The protective effect was found with a daily intake of one hundred micrograms of folic acid and was not found with vitamins other than folic acid.

Evidence of nutritional deficiency based on dietary recall is subject to bias and inaccuracies. A more direct and objective measure of nutritional status was needed to strengthen the evidence. Blood levels of folic acid are difficult to interpret, but biochemical evidence was soon forthcoming in that mothers who had babies with spina bifida had lower red blood cell folic acid concentration than did mothers in a control group.

This evidence implicating folic acid is very exciting. It is known, for

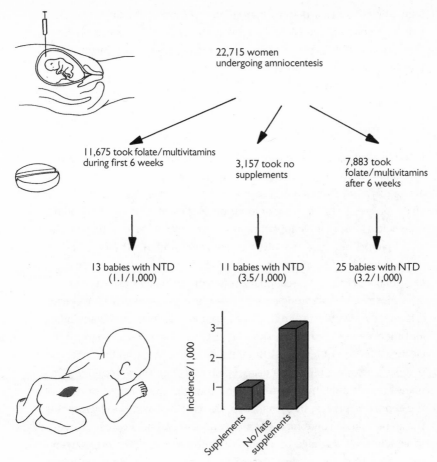

22,715 women
undergoing amniocentesis

11,675 took folate/multivitamins
during first 6 weeks

3,157 took no
supplements

7,883 took
folate/multivitamins
after 6 weeks

13 babies with NTD
(1.1/1,000)

11 babies with NTD
(3.5/1,000)

25 babies with NTD
(3.2/1,000)

Incidence/1,000

Supplements

No/late
supplements

Figure 3.2. A prospective study implicating folate supplementation in the prevention of neural tube defects (NTD). The incidence of spina bifida among those women who took supplements during the first six weeks was less than a third of the other groups (data from Milunsky et al. 1989).

example, that folic acid is an essential nutrient that plays a key role in metabolism. Moreover, the need for adequate folic acid is likely to be most critical during times of rapid cell division and migration, such as the period of neural tube formation in the embryo. There is also evidence from animal experiments in which folic acid deficiency or the use of aminopterin, a folic acid antagonist, was found to cause a variety of central nervous system malformations. Several different lines of research are pointing toward folic acid deficiency. Not only is there evidence of an association between low folic acid intake in early pregnancy and spina bifida, but there is also an emerging appreciation of the mechanism involved. A cohesive theory of the etiology of neural tube defects is on the horizon, one that explains what causal factors are responsible and how they lead to the malformations. Surely such an understanding should lead to the prevention of spina bifida?

Is Prevention Possible?

Before we can answer the question of whether spina bifida can be prevented, we need to distinguish between primary prevention and secondary prevention. Primary prevention entails intervening to prevent the chain of events in early embryonic development that leads to neural tube defects from ever happening in the first place—to alter those nutritional factors (and possibly other factors) that underlie the birth defect. The eradication of smallpox through vaccination was a dramatic example of primary prevention. Secondary prevention involves an intervention after those early embryologic events have already taken place. Of course, it is already possible and indeed commonplace to "prevent" spina bifida and anencephaly secondarily through pregnancy screening programs and elective abortion of fetuses. Although a satisfactory option for some, this practice carries with it a great deal of pain and anguish. It would be a dramatic breakthrough indeed to develop a technique that arrests or reverses the abnormal process in the embryo, thereby improving or even curing the spina bifida. There have been advances in the field of fetal surgery, in which surgeons have been able to shunt fetuses with severe hydrocephalus, but it is clear that such efforts have so far not led to improved outcomes. Unfortunately, therapeutic techniques directed at the tiny embryo seem a long way off.

On the other hand, knowing what we know about the likely nutritional causes of neural tube defects, there is every reason to consider that the primary prevention of most cases of spina bifida is a realistic objective and one that is not far out of our grasp. In a more recent study, the U.K. Multicenter Trial (Smithells 1991), a large number of women who had previously had a baby or fetus with a neural tube defect were contacted and urged to take a multivitamin–folic acid tablet three times a day around the time of conception and through the first trimester. Some took the tablets as suggested, others did not. Twenty-four of 519 women who did not take the supplements had a second neural tube defect pregnancy. Only 3 of 454 women who took the tablets as suggested and 0 of 114 who were felt to be partially supplemented had recurrences of neural tube defects (Figure 3.3).

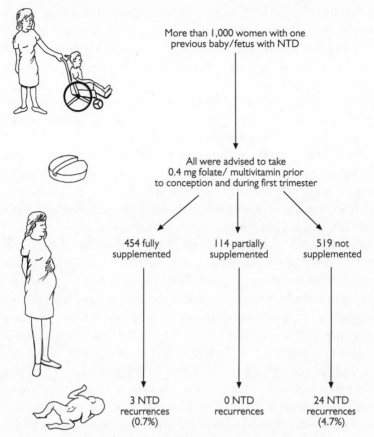

More than 1,000 women with one
previous baby/fetus with NTD

All were advised to take
0.4 mg folate/ multivitamin prior
to conception and during first trimester

| 454 fully supplemented | 114 partially supplemented | 519 not supplemented |

| 3 NTD recurrences (0.7%) | 0 NTD recurrences | 24 NTD recurrences (4.7%) |

Figure 3.3. The prevention of spina bifida. In the U.K. Multicenter Trial (Smithells 1991) there were dramatically fewer recurrences of spina bifida among women who were fully supplemented with 0.4 mg of folic acid.

The United Kingdom Medical Research Council (MRC) trial of vitamin supplementation (1991) also clearly shows a protective effect of 4 milligrams of folic acid daily around conception and into early pregnancy. The recurrence rate was about 1 percent in mothers taking folic acid and 3.5 percent in those not receiving it. There was no protective effect for other vitamins. Very similar results were obtained in a study in Cuba. The consistency of the findings is remarkable.

In 1992, the results of a Hungarian study were published in the *New England Journal of Medicine* (Czeizel and Dudas 1992). This was a randomized, controlled trial of multivitamin supplements given at least one month before conception until the end of the first trimester. Women planning a pregnancy were randomized to take either a multivitamin plus 0.8 milligrams of folic acid or a trace element supplement without folic acid. There were six cases of neural tube defect in the babies of the trace element group, compared with none in the vitamin–folic acid group. Unlike the previous studies, this study examined the incidence of first-time spina bifida, rather than recurrences in women who had already had one such pregnancy, and showed a clear protective effect.

The Centers for Disease Control (CDC) in Atlanta is currently involved in an intervention study in China, which will be on a very large scale and which is likely to provide still more definitive answers. The results of this enormous study are eagerly awaited. But while we wait, what are the public health implications of the evidence that already exists?

Certainly, it is beyond doubt that women who have already had a neural tube defect pregnancy should be on folic acid supplements totaling at least 4 milligrams per day prior to and following conception. It would also be prudent for women who have a family history of spina bifida to take folic acid supplements. Moreover, the time has come when we should be recommending 0.4 milligrams daily folic acid supplementation to all women who are trying to conceive. Because many women in this country do not receive early prenatal care or do not know they are pregnant until two or three months into their pregnancies, the most sensible means of ensuring adequate folic acid intake among women in the childbearing years is to fortify staple foods such as bread, cereals, and pasta. This approach is used in infants, in whom iron deficiency is prevented through the enrichment of formula and cereals. It would be a safe and inexpensive public health measure and could potentially prevent the occurrence of spina bifida for a large number of families. The CDC estimates that up to 75 percent of cases of spina bifida may be preventable by folic acid supplementation, which is scheduled to become effective in January 1997.

THE ROLE OF GENETICS

Of course, the nutritional hypothesis is not the whole story. As in most conditions in medicine, there are probably a number of different causes of spina bifida. For some children, the problem may have been related to folic acid deficiency. For some, other factors may have been operating to interfere with neural tube closure. Certainly, evidence indicates that thoracic-level spina bifida differs from lumbar-level spina bifida in several interesting ways. The sex ratio, for example, is different: more females have thoracic spina bifida than do males. Thoracic spina bifida may be significantly more common in whites than in African Americans (Greene et al. 1991). Neither of these phenomena is true in lumbar spina bifida. Thoracic spina bifida is also associated with other midline defects, including multiple neural tube defects. One child I know has thoracic spina bifida, as well as an encephalocele and a cervical meningocele, for example. These various associations point to the likelihood of a genetic susceptibility to neural tube defects, that some inherited genes make the developing embryo vulnerable in some way to these abnormalities. In a small minority of cases of spina bifida, there are identifiable chromosomal abnormalities, such as a ring chromosome, a deletion of part of a chromosome, or a trisomy (an extra chromosome). However, there are no consistent patterns, and in any case, most subtle genetic abnormalities are not evident on regular chromosome studies. At this point, we have not identified specific genes responsible for spina bifida, but studies in this area are underway involving families with more than one child with spina bifida.

OTHER CLUES AND POSSIBILITIES

In the laboratory, it is possible to alter the environment of the embryo in various ways in an effort to learn more about birth defects. This is the study of teratogenesis. There are many teratogenic substances that can produce neural tube defects; thus the timing of the insult is probably more important than the nature of the insult itself. However, one substance that deserves special mention is Agent Orange, a defoliant that was used extensively in the Vietnam War. Many members of the U.S. armed forces were exposed to Agent Orange, and in the years that followed, it became increasingly evident that these individuals were experiencing diverse health problems. There were also some reports of a higher-than-expected incidence of birth defects, including spina bifida, among their offspring. A class action suit was brought against the armed forces and the manufacturers of Agent Orange, and funds from this settlement were set aside for treatment of conditions among Vietnam veterans that may be associated with this substance. It is currently thought that Agent Orange did not actually cause cases of spina bifida, but it is important to remember that these funds may be available to assist eligible families.

Another line of research that is turning up some interesting information is that of placental metabolism. Placental cells are partially derived from the embryo itself, so that abnormal placental metabolism may reflect abnormal metabolism of fetal cells. There is some evidence that the cells in the placentae of babies with neural tube defects show abnormal metabolism of folic acid.

Some babies with thoracic spina bifida have unusual rib malformations and congenital scoliosis, which suggests that the developing embryo had an abnormality of the blood vessels supplying nutrients to those areas. This hypothesized vascular cause of spina bifida may represent an unusual form of spina bifida.

There is one last note that is a little provocative, although completely unsubstantiated at this point. In a recently published survey from Louisiana, an unexpected association was found between neural tube defects and hot baths! Women who, in early pregnancy, had bathed in hot tubs or Jacuzzis where the water was hot enough to make their skin red when they emerged from the water, were more likely to have had an affected fetus (Sandford, Kissling, and Joubert 1992). The survey was very extensive, and so it is quite possible that this apparent association just arose by chance. But there may be some theoretical basis to it, because it is known that hyperthermia in early pregnancy can interfere with the development of mammalian embryos. Evidence from retrospective studies also links neural tube defects to infections with fever in early pregnancy. The possibility that prolonged hot baths or Jacuzzis that are hot enough to raise significantly the body temperature might adversely affect the embryo is intriguing and requires further research.

PRENATAL SCREENING FOR NEURAL TUBE DEFECTS

Women who have already had one fetus with a neural tube defect have a 2 percent recurrence risk—that is, one in fifty pregnancies would be likely to result in a second fetus with a neural tube defect. However, around 95 percent of cases of spina bifida arise in families with no prior history of neural tube defects. Any effort to screen for this condition prenatally should therefore be aimed at all pregnant women, not just those who, by virtue of a previous affected fetus, are at increased risk.

In 1972, Brock and Sutcliffe reported the association between increased amounts of alpha-fetoprotein in amniotic fluid and neural tube defects. The following year, it was demonstrated that this substance was often elevated in the mother's blood under these circumstances. This breakthrough opened the door to maternal serum alpha-fetoprotein screening as a screening procedure for the entire population of pregnant women.

Of course, things are never as simple as they sound. For a start, the levels of this substance change continuously during the second trimester of pregnancy. Screening before fifteen weeks is very unreliable. There is a narrow window of opportunity, because screening between nineteen and twenty-one weeks allows very little time for decision making about the possibility of therapeutic abortion. Most screening programs therefore offer screening to women between fifteen and twenty weeks of gestation. Next, the assay is demanding and requires great precision. The cutoff points have to be carefully established, and little difference often exists between a normal test and an abnormal one. Hence, a normal test doesn't guarantee a normal baby. The sensitivity of the screening blood test is approximately 80 percent—that is, it should pick up eight out of ten fetuses with a neural tube defect. An abnormally elevated test does not necessarily mean the baby has a neural tube defect. Elevated levels can also result from underestimated gestational age, twins, or bleeding. The specificity of the initial screen is probably around 40 percent, so that four out of ten elevated tests will actually be confirmed to be neural tube defects. For this reason, many screening programs employ a second blood test and proceed to ultrasound only if this too is elevated. In some circumstances, amniocentesis may be helpful for measurement of alpha-fetoprotein and possibly for chromosome analysis. All these steps have to be completed in a maximum of four weeks if termination of pregnancy is to be considered an option (Figure 3.4).

In addition to the exacting standards required of the alpha-fetoprotein laboratory, a comprehensive screening program requires that the following criteria be met: First, obstetricians and other health professionals need to understand the objectives of screening and testing, the importance of the timing of tests, and the need for follow-up procedures and counseling. Second, adequate facilities and experienced professionals must be available to follow up with counseling, high-resolution ultrasound, and amniocentesis. Third, careful attention must be paid to education and informed consent of the mother at every step. Some women may not want to be confronted with the dilemma posed by an abnormal test result, and participation in screening should be voluntary. It is an important responsibility of the provider, however, to go to great lengths to explain, educate, and encourage participation. The overriding concern and goal of the screening program should be to provide women and couples with the information they need to make their decisions.

In my own clinical practice, the obstetricians and counselors who provide services for the University of North Carolina Alpha-Fetoprotein Screening Program know that I am available as an additional resource for women who are carrying a fetus with diagnosed spina bifida. Because

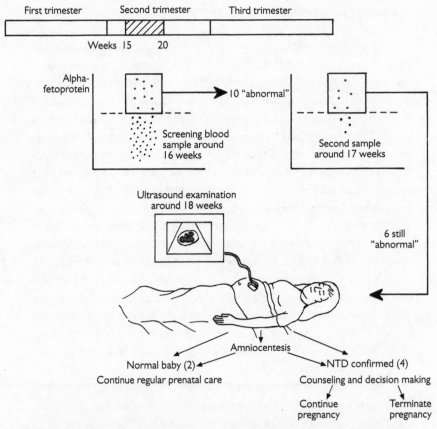

Figure 3.4. Steps and decision making in screening programs for neural tube defects. Among one thousand women screened, ten may have an elevated blood alpha-fetoprotein (AFP) level. Of these, only four NTDs are later confirmed by ultrasound and/or amniocentesis.

time is of the essence in decision making regarding a pregnancy that may already be at around nineteen or twenty weeks, I will take such referrals at short notice and arrange to meet the parent(s). My role at such a meeting is to explore with them their knowledge of spina bifida and their attitudes and fears about having a child with a chronic illness or disability. Often, in spite of pamphlets about spina bifida and educational efforts by others, parents have misconceptions about the condition. Some have thought that the initial operation to close the defect would lead to completely normal function. Others have understood that the presence of hydrocephalus indicated that the baby would never learn to read or write. Others base their impressions on one individual with spina bifida, perhaps a neighbor's child, a distant relative, or an adult in their community. It is not uncommon that other counselors have attempted to predict the unpredictable or to present a "worst case" scenario to the parents-to-be. The early appearance of hydrocephalus is sometimes perceived by obstetricians and others as a grim sign, an indicator that the fetus's brain is severely affected and that the neurologic and cognitive outcome is bleak. This is not clearly the case, as we shall see in Chapter 4, and it is important that parents understand that various outcomes exist and that only time will tell. How to proceed is a lonely and painful decision, one I can't make for them. I can only tell them that whatever decision they choose to make is the right decision for them.

For those parents-to-be who decide to go ahead with the pregnancy, a prenatal meeting with an expert in spina bifida can be very helpful. There may also be an opportunity to meet the members of the health care team and to learn about the clinic. I have found it especially helpful to arrange such meetings on a clinic day, which affords the opportunity, if the mother or couple is emotionally ready for this experience, to come to the clinic with me and to meet another family that grappled with these same problems not long ago. Of course, one has to be judicious in making the appropriate match, both in terms of the severity and nature of the child's spina bifida and also the parents' background. I have been so impressed with the value of such encounters. It serves to communicate directly to the parents-to-be that there is a future, a light at the end of the tunnel. They get to see schoolchildren, kids with personalities and a sense of humor, and they see families that are coping. It can be uplifting and energizing, dispelling fears and misconceptions that repeatedly haunt their imaginations. Such is my fervent belief in the power of parent-to-parent contact that I have asked parents to help me write this book by sharing their personal stories and offering advice based on their real-life experiences. These very special sections are at the end of most of the following chapters.

THE FUTURE OF IN UTERO SURGERY

With the advent of high-resolution ultrasound scanning, we have become familiar with clearer and clearer images of fetuses kicking, moving, stretching, and sucking. Almost every organ in the fetus can be visualized, so that it has become possible to examine the movements of the valves of the fetus's beating heart and the contraction of the bladder during urination, for example. This technology has allowed specialists to go beyond diagnosis of the fetal patient and to attempt medical and surgical treatments. Today, it is possible for catheters to be placed in umbilical blood vessels to give blood transfusions, obstructed urinary tracts to be drained, or fluid to be withdrawn from chest or abdominal cavities. A few fetuses have even been delivered to undergo intricate surgery and then carefully returned to the womb to continue development!

The most challenging of problems are those of the central nervous system. Researchers have grappled with the question of the best treatment options for fetal hydrocephalus that is increasing rapidly on serial ultrasound scans. When this occurs in the third trimester, at around thirty to thirty-three weeks, the option of early delivery can be considered if the baby is considered to be sufficiently mature. When the fetus is in the second trimester, however, the question of intrauterine surgery may be raised. The question is particularly vexing because no clear relationship exists between the extent of fetal hydrocephalus and subsequent neurologic outcome.

In 1981, the first procedure to drain hydrocephalus in a human fetus was performed. Subsequently, the technique of insertion of ventriculo-amniotic shunts was developed, whereby a fine catheter is placed under ultrasound control into the fetus's dilated ventricles, thus allowing the CSF to drain into the amniotic fluid. Although a simple idea, the procedure was fraught with difficulty. Complications included dislodgement of the shunt, infections, and premature delivery. The mortality rate of the procedure was about 25 percent. For the survivors, it is not certain that the surgery improved their outcome. The procedure has now largely been suspended and is no longer an option. Research in the next decade, however, may point the way to treatments that are relatively safe and effective, but these will have to be carefully evaluated before they become widely available. It is the history of medical innovations that new techniques are initially greeted with great enthusiasm, then pessimistically dismissed, and finally resurrected and improved. I anticipate that some children in the twenty-first century will have been very successfully treated before they were ever born!

CHAPTER 4

Pregnancy and Childbirth

I received a telephone call from the obstetrician in the prenatal diagnosis clinic. She wanted to refer a young couple, Mr. and Mrs. K., who had just received a diagnosis of spina bifida. This was their first pregnancy. Mrs. K. had a raised AFP, and the ultrasound had confirmed their worst fears. At seventeen weeks of gestation, the female fetus appeared to have a large lumbar myelomeningocele and hydrocephalus. They had been told that the hydrocephalus was a bad sign.

When I saw them the next day, they were composed and asked many questions about spina bifida and the implications of the scan results. I could not be very specific in my answers and tried to give them a likely range of possibilities. Mr. K. was most concerned about whether she would walk, run, and play. Mrs. K. cried and indicated that she mostly feared that her daughter would never learn to talk because of the hydrocephalus. I attempted to draw them out regarding their thoughts on continuing or terminating the pregnancy, stressing that the choice was theirs and whichever they chose was the right choice for them. They were a little guarded, but I sensed that Mrs. K. was inclined to continue, drawing on her trust in God, whereas Mr. K. was more ambivalent. They asked me if they could visit the clinic to see some children with spina bifida and their parents, but I was not comfortable with setting up a situation where they might be unduly influenced by other parents.

The next day, Mr. K. called me to say they had decided to continue the pregnancy. I made arrangements for them to come to clinic the following week. They met some of the other clinic staff, and we introduced them to another family. They spent an hour together in private and came out smiling and obviously more secure in their decision than I had seen them previously.

PREPARING FOR ARRIVAL

There are some valuable lessons for us all here. What a strange phrase it is "to receive a diagnosis." Normally, we receive gifts, or at the very least, we know or we can see what it is we are receiving. To receive a diagnosis of a birth defect in an unborn child is a terrifying process because the recipient is almost always in the dark and lacking in information. When we are in the dark our fears are amplified by our imaginations. Parents in this situation may feel overwhelmed with shock, anxiety, and helplessness. Couples may be in very different spaces psychologically. One may be angry and full of denial, whereas the other may be in need of comfort and support. They may have private and personal fears or preoccupations that they find difficult to share, such that communication between them is strained. It is a difficult time to absorb new information or even to frame the questions to ask.

Doctors too find these situations very difficult to handle, and it is almost impossible to say the right thing. No wonder so many parents have bad memories of these encounters. There is a wealth of information about this topic from the doctor's perspective (Klein 1993). Some of the common pitfalls include giving a barrage of clinical information which is not understood and which is perceived as cold or "talking at" the parents-to-be. Sometimes, in a well-meaning attempt to provide comfort and ease the suffering, we doctors may continually offer words of encouragement or paint things in a rosy light. Perhaps the most appropriate path is to provide a little information and allow parents their natural feelings of grief, anger, and despair. Often they need time alone, and the doctor should respect this need and make arrangements to continue the informational process later.

It is crucial for us doctors not to go out on a limb and make predictions with any degree of certainty, for these will almost surely come back to haunt us. It is far better to discuss a realistic range. Will she walk? In all probability, she will need help to walk, and this is likely to involve bracing and orthopedic surgery. Maybe she will do better in a wheelchair when she is older. Will he talk? Unless there is some very serious complication, he will talk, and he will probably begin talking at the usual time. Will she be able to go to a regular school? Many children with spina bifida have learning problems, and she may need some special help at school. The clinician must remember that "I don't know" is sometimes the most honest and even the most helpful answer to some of these very challenging questions.

The doctor has a crucial responsibility to tease out and adjust misconceptions. Among the most common of these is the deterministic notion that early hydrocephalus spells a poor outcome. I have seen many children born with moderate or severe hydrocephalus who do just as well as some with minimal hydrocephalus. Again, the unpredictability of cognitive and learning outcomes should be stressed. Another common misconception surrounds the use of the term "mental retardation," which is frequently used by well-meaning clinicians who don't realize how differently some people interpret the term. Many parents think of the very severe end of the spectrum of mental retardation when they hear the term, and such an image does not fit well with the typical range of cognition and behavior among children with spina bifida. They may assume that their child will always be dependent on them. It may be helpful to point out that many people with mild mental retardation can read, learn, find productive employment, travel, fall in love, and have children. They may achieve considerable independence in a society that is becoming increasingly diverse and conscious of disability. Fulfillment and a sense of mastery flow from independence. For nondisabled children, we often take their progress toward independence for granted, whereas parents of successful and fulfilled children with spina bifida have told me and shown me that they have had to be proactive in promoting independence from a very early age. Doctors can help parents to lay the groundwork for future independence by encouraging them to think about these issues.

THINGS TO DO IN PREGNANCY

The most crucial thing for an expectant mother to do is to obtain good prenatal care. This should be with an obstetrician whom you trust, one who will keep a close eye on you and also provide extra emotional support. The growth and development of the fetus will need to be monitored, especially for the detection of rapidly progressive hydrocephalus. This will entail the use of ultrasound examinations. These tests are completely harmless and give the obstetrician valuable information about the best way to manage your pregnancy (Figure 4.1).

The ultrasound examination gives the doctor pretty good views of the spine, so that the position of the myelomeningocele can be determined. In the hands of a skilled ultrasound specialist, it may be possible to predict likely muscle function. Commonly, a pregnant woman will feel falsely reassured when she observes a very active fetus on ultrasound, thinking that

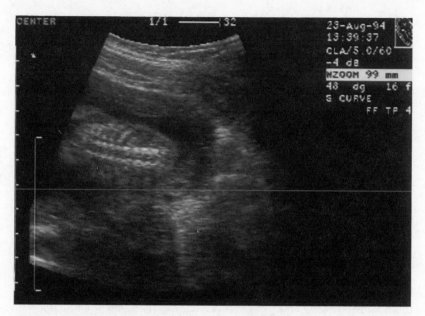

Figure 4.1. The ultrasound examination shows details of the spine as well as the presence of hydrocephalus.

her baby will not have significant paralysis. Unfortunately, the presence of such movements on ultrasound does not reliably predict that the degree of paralysis will be mild.

The degree of hydrocephalus can be quite accurately assessed using ultrasound examination. If the hydrocephalus is stable and not extreme, this is a reassuring sign that the growth and development of the brain is not being compromised. Under these circumstances, it would be normal practice to allow the fetus to remain in the safest environment, namely, the uterus. If the hydrocephalus is severe or progressing rapidly, however, this may cause pressure on the brain, affecting its development. Under these circumstances, the safest option may be to deliver the baby prematurely to place a shunt and relieve the CSF pressure after birth. Naturally, the risks of prematurity will have to be balanced against the risks of allowing the hydrocephalus to progress. The most important risk of prematurity is that the lungs will be immature and the baby will develop respiratory distress syndrome (RDS) and need respiratory support, including a ventilator and oxygen. Lung maturity of the fetus can be assessed by testing a sample of amniotic fluid via amniocentesis. It is usually possible to gauge the risk of complications of prematurity in this way. Furthermore, the use of steroids before delivery can sometimes enhance fetal lung maturity sufficiently to reduce the risk of immature lung development. Most babies of thirty-three weeks' gestation can avoid RDS, whereas the vast majority of babies under thirty weeks have RDS. Generally, the more premature babies have more severe lung disease; thus the likelihood of survival of babies under twenty-five to twenty-six weeks is very low. Although it is ideal to delay delivery until after thirty-three weeks, the severity of the hydrocephalus may force an early delivery.

The diagnosis of a birth defect is such an important event that the usual prenatal care issues are sometimes overlooked. These crucial aspects of prenatal care include gaining the appropriate amount of weight, taking vitamins, getting regular exercise, and discussing sexuality. Rest, relaxation, and healthy habits are as important for the mother of a fetus with spina bifida as they are for any other pregnant woman.

Caution should be exercised with the use of over-the-counter and prescription medicines, especially as the effects of these on hydrocephalus are simply not known. If there is any doubt at all, consult your physician.

DELIVERY

Delivery should be carried out in a medical center where there is expert neonatal intensive care and an experienced neurosurgeon. It makes no sense to deliver the baby in a hospital that lacks these facilities and then have to transport the baby to another hospital. Transport of a sick newborn presents many problems, not the least of which is the anxiety on the part of the parents who are left behind. It is far more sensible to transport the baby in the comfort and safety of the womb prior to delivery. It is advisable to plan ahead in case premature labor starts.

Labor is a lot of work and often a stressful experience for a baby in the best of circumstances. The contractions of the uterus are extremely strong and exert pressure on the baby's body. For the baby with spina bifida and hydrocephalus, the stress of labor and vaginal delivery may be increased. Often the baby is in breech presentation because of the leg paralysis, and this position increases the risk of complications. The enlarged head may not engage easily, or if engaged, it may get stuck in the birth canal. Moreover, the unprotected neural elements of the myelomeningocele are subject to pressure and shearing forces in the process. It is not uncommon for a previously intact sac to rupture, leaving the spinal cord directly exposed to trauma and infection. For these reasons, many centers recommend cesarian section before the onset of labor for delivery of babies known to have myelomeningocele. Usually, this is scheduled for around thirty-five weeks' gestation. In one follow-up study of babies delivered by cesarian section without labor, the infants had less-severe paralysis than did those delivered vaginally or by cesarian section after labor. There is some controversy about this issue, however, and the evidence is not certain. Until such evidence is available, some circumstances may exist in which vaginal delivery is appropriate.

INFORMATION GATHERING

Your pregnancy is a valuable time to find out more about spina bifida so that you know what to expect and can be better prepared. If you are married, involve your husband. If not, request the support of your boyfriend, girlfriend, or trusted family member as you go about gathering information. Your obstetrician may be helpful in putting you in touch with a genetics counselor, pediatrician, nurse, or another professional who is knowledgeable about the condition.

The Spina Bifida Association of America (SBAA) will be a valuable resource for you and will continue to be a resource for life. As a nonprofit voluntary association interested in health care, the SBAA is dedicated to making the public as well as professional and governmental agencies more aware of spina bifida and to helping parents help their children. There are thousands of members, parents like you who may have been through similar experiences. A chapter of SBAA may be found in almost every state. (See the Appendix for a list of state and local chapters as well as selected international Spina Bifida Associations.) Other countries have similar groups, networks, and associations. In the United Kingdom, the Association for Spina Bifida and Hydrocephalus (ASBAH) has long been active in providing education and support to families of children with spina bifida and hydrocephalus. In Canada and in Australia, there are parent associations in every province. Such agencies also produce newsletters and publications that can be very informative. Through agencies such as these, you should be able to obtain information about clinics that provide care and expertise in the management of spina bifida. If you feel ready for this, such information can also be helpful. Be cautious about going to the local library and looking up information in old medical books. Some of what you may read there is very out-of-date and may not give you a true picture of what to expect.

As you gather information, remember to keep things in perspective and keep your life in balance. Take care of yourself, and take care of your relationships. Don't let this quest for information become all-consuming.

Remember that others may not be as ready to face this as you are and that they may need a lot of reassurance. Knowledge is important, but it is only a part of what you will need in the months and years to come. Love and support are also vital ingredients!

Making the Right Choice for Health Care

The SBAA and the contacts that you make locally through the SBAA may be helpful in suggesting certain clinics or professionals who have expertise in spina bifida. Specialized multidisciplinary clinics, where your child will be able to receive comprehensive care by a team of doctors and allied health professionals, are widely distributed in most countries and in most of the United States. Such clinics offer several advantages to families. The services are coordinated, so that you will periodically get the health care and advice you need at one visit, rather than having to bounce around from clinic to clinic, appointment to appointment, and doctor to doctor. Clinics such as these are not all exactly alike, and the makeup of the team may vary according to the availability, interests, and strengths of the professionals involved. Typically, the teams consist of a neurosurgeon, orthopedic surgeon, urologist, pediatrician, nurse, physical therapist, orthotics specialist, and occupational therapist. Sometimes, a psychologist and/or a social worker may be involved. In some centers, specialists in physical medicine and rehabilitation are important team members. It may seem that such an enormous team is unnecessary and inefficient and that visits to such a clinic might last a week! In reality, it is seldom necessary to see all members of the team, and the visits should be structured to address your concerns as efficiently as possible. Remember that you can make active choices in health care in order to meet your specific needs.

Finding the right health care services may be very straightforward. There may be one such team at a medical center near you and no other options in your area. If, on the other hand, there is more than one option or if the only such team is a great distance away, seek advice from parents and professionals in your community.

One important health care issue that is often forgotten is primary care. Your baby with spina bifida is going to get colds, ear infections, rashes, and a host of childhood ailments, just like other children, and will also require immunizations and well-child care. And you may need advice about nutrition, child rearing, and behavioral issues. For all these important needs, a general practitioner, family doctor, or pediatrician should be found in your community. Special experience in spina bifida is not important, because your baby will in most respects be a "normal" baby, and you will have access to specialists if and when you need them.

Partnerships with Professionals

This section is written for both parents and professionals, in an effort to encourage the kind of constructive, trusting relationships between us that will lead to mutual participation in family-centered care and decision making. Parents are experts about their child and can serve as teachers and partners to professionals. This view is clearly articulated in Public Law 99-457, the federal legislation regarding early intervention and family-based service planning for infants and toddlers with disabilities (see Chapter 11). In the past, parents were usually expected to be passive and to defer to the physician's judgment. Outspoken mothers of children with disabilities were (and often still are) viewed as demanding, difficult, and even hostile. Fortunately, growing experience in the management of chronic conditions in childhood has led to the growth of parent-professional partnerships. The partnership concept and the model of mutual participation are most appropriate for chronic conditions such as spina bifida because the doctor, patient, and family work together toward mutual goals. The model is most likely to be successful when there is a common understanding of the problems and a common plan of management. From a practical perspective, this means that health care is likely to be most effective when the parents and professionals are actively learning from each other how best to help the child.

Parents, you should know that doctors want to hear your concerns and appreciate your active participation. Keep records and write a list of your questions or concerns. Some of the most satisfying, positive, and therapeutic doctor-patient relationships have been with parents who are assertive and knowledgeable.

Doctors, you should know that studies have demonstrated improved compliance in treatment regimens among families who feel themselves to be mutual participants in the treatment plans. Successful health outcomes are more likely if parents feel respected and praised. The settings of clinical encounters should be conducive to open communication and active give-and-take of information among adults of equal status. A helpful technique is to inquire about parental observations of the child's development and behavior. This process enables the doctor to explore parental expectations and to link the parental observations with specific clinical findings. In discussing relevant clinical issues, doctors will want to avoid and to clarify mystifying jargon and medical terminology. When parents express their frustrations, doubts, or negative feelings, it is important for the doctor to convey understanding, empathy, and support. Parents tend to suppress these feelings in clinical encounters, which requires a lot of psychic energy. By providing the parent(s) an opportunity to express such feelings to you and, if applicable, to each other, some of this energy is released for more constructive efforts to deal with the concerns at hand. If there are problems with noncompliance, these may well stem from differing perspectives and priorities between parents and doctors. To get onto similar wavelengths and influence care in positive ways, we need to be thinking in terms of functional outcomes and quality of life, not just medical or technical outcomes.

PARENT-TO-PARENT

There are questions that will arise concerning day-to-day issues and minor problems, which the professionals you have identified just won't be able to answer. They may not have the benefit of the experience of coping with some of these issues, and their advice may not always be practical. Who better to give you practical advice than another parent who has been where you are, who has learned from mistakes, and who wants to share some of this experience with you? Your SBAA chapter or spina bifida clinic may suggest a family for you to contact. Alternatively, there may be meetings of the parent group periodically. If possible, both parents-to-be should be involved in these parent-to-parent contacts: this is a shared learning experience that you should go through together.

CHAPTER 5

The Newborn Baby

The birth of a baby is a human experience unparalleled in its drama and intensity. Although the management of labor and delivery in hospitals has undergone some rehumanization during recent years, the medical technology can often be intimidating to parents. This is especially true with babies who are known to have problems that are going to require special care, because there is an air of expectant urgency in the delivery room as the medical team stands by ready for action! A visit to the labor and delivery unit can help prepare parents for the experience. I hope this chapter will also be helpful to expectant parents of a baby with spina bifida.

The chapter begins with a discussion of important issues about the behavior and development of the newborn baby, followed by a section on habilitation issues, especially feeding. Next, many aspects of the medical care of the newborn baby with spina bifida are described to familiarize the reader with some of the things that commonly occur. The chapter also contains up-to-date medical information that I hope will be of interest to physicians, nurses, and other health care professionals who care for babies with spina bifida.

DEVELOPMENTAL ISSUES

Observing Your Baby's Development

In the eyes of a parent, a marvelous transformation occurs after a baby with spina bifida is born. Before delivery and in the early days of intense concern about closure, shunting, and other medical issues, the focus is on the problems and hazards. As anxiety decreases, a parent is able to regard and observe the baby more closely, in the minutest detail, and come to know him or her as a unique new individual. Imperceptibly, the focus changes from pathology to personality, and the little one becomes a "normal" baby (who happens to have spina bifida). This new focus brings with it the appreciation of nuances of development and temperament, so that parent and baby come to know and experience each other in ever increasing richness. The transactions that take place during these early days are very important for attachment and bonding and lay the foundations for subsequent relationships.

Babies are perfectly adapted to communicate with their mothers and fathers. Although they are so utterly dependent on parents for feeding, carrying, and comforting, they are certainly not passive. They elicit help and love from their caregivers, using cues and signals that are almost guaranteed to get results. They love to look at the human face and prefer to gaze into an adult's eyes than at any other stimulus. Notice how your baby is able to sustain a quiet, alert state while staring intently into your eyes. Extraneous movements of little arms and hands are stilled, and even breathing quiets as his eyes study your face. When you talk softly to your baby, observe how he listens, and when you stop talking, see how he starts to move, fuss, or cry to get you to talk again! By the age of one month, not only is your baby fixing her gaze, but she is also following you with her eyes as you move slowly in her field of vision. Observe how her hands move, the way her fingers open to allow her to explore her world, holding your finger or touching your face or breast as you feed her.

Figure 5.1 shows some of the key developmental milestones of newborns and babies up to two months of age. These are shown not to measure a baby's level of development but to illustrate the range of special competencies of the young human infant. By observing these and other developmental skills in your baby, you will grow in your appreciation and wonder at how well put together he is! In so doing, you will be focusing on his strengths and abilities, rather than on potential disabilities. This orientation is extremely important and will become even more so later on.

Of course, not all babies are the same. Many parents of two children will tell you how different they are. Although two siblings may share similar genetic backgrounds and environments, they come into this world with different characteristics, different patterns of behavior, and different ways of interacting. This is what is meant by the term "temperament" in infants. These individual differences are evident even in tiny infants, and there is a moderate degree of continuity, so that the same behavioral style may be evident across the years. Some babies are especially placid, calm, and easygoing. As infants, they may be likely to settle easily, and later they may seem to pass through the "terrible twos" with few temper tantrums or power struggles. Other babies are highly charged, erratic in schedules,

Aspects of development	One week	Four weeks	Eight weeks
Sensory	Follows face horizontally	Tracks parent's movement	Visual acuity much increased
	Turns to face	Distinguishes parent's voice	Turns smoothly to localize sounds
	Startles to loud sound		
	Orients toward mother's smell		
	Sucks breast milk more vigorously		
Sleep/wake cycles	Begins to develop cycles	Has much more regular cycles	Has established day-night rhythm
	Brief quiet-alert times	Longer quiet-alert times	
Motor	Moves arms jerkily	Moves arms more smoothly	Wiggles when looking at object
		Regards own hand	May swipe at objects in reach
Social	Preferentially looks at face	May smile in response	Smiles to elicit response
		Carefully scans faces	
		Communicates by crying and via body language	
Self-soothing	Can be calmed by parent	Able to turn away actively	Has increased periods of fussiness, colic
	Responds to rocking	Develops predictable response to rocking, soothing, feeding	

Figure 5.1. Developmental milestones of early infancy (from birth to two months)

and irritable. As they get older they may be more likely to have sleep difficulties and temper tantrums. Broadly speaking, there are three patterns of temperament (although many babies do not fit neatly into one group, sharing attributes from two or three groups). These styles of temperament have been termed "easy," "slow to warm up," and "difficult." The chief characteristics of these three groups are given in Figure 5.2. Get to know your baby's temperament. How does she make her needs known to you? How does she respond to you? How easily does she adapt to changes?

Easy	Slow to warm up	Difficult
Regular, predictable	Some irregularity	Irregular, unpredictable
Positive, smiling	Often negative in response	Negative, irritable
Adapts easily to change	Adapts with some difficulty to transitions	Adapts poorly to change
Enjoys new stimuli	Is slow to warm up, responds tentatively	Withdraws from new stimuli, shows intense reactions

Figure 5.2. Temperament characteristics

HABILITATION ISSUES

Feeding and Feeding Difficulties

For all newborn babies, breast-feeding has certain advantages. Breast milk has an excellent balance of protein, vitamins, and minerals and also provides immunological protection against infection. Several safe and nutritionally balanced infant formulas are a suitable alternative for those mothers who stop breast-feeding or decide to bottle-feed.

Most newborn babies will feed about two or three ounces of milk at each feed and will want to feed six or more times a day. At five to six weeks old, the baby will likely be taking five or six ounces five or six times a day. By three or four months of age, he may be up to seven or eight ounces, and the number of feedings, down to four or five. If you are lucky, he will be sleeping through the night. If he habitually awakens and cries at night at around four months of age, remember that his growing body no longer needs that 2:00 A.M. feed. He probably just likes it and enjoys your company. See if you can soothe him back to sleep, or give him a little water in the bottle instead.

Breast milk or formula is the only food that the baby needs until around four months of age. There is a temptation to start solid foods early, sometimes in an effort to "satisfy" a baby who demands to be fed frequently (even in the early hours of the morning). Starting solid foods too early and giving too much of them can cause obesity, and obese babies usually become obese toddlers. Nobody likes to put young children on a diet, and it is hard for a parent or a doting grandparent to deny food to a child. We will return to prevention of obesity in subsequent chapters, for obesity is very common and entirely preventable in children with spina bifida. The first step, therefore, is to avoid starting solid foods before four months of age.

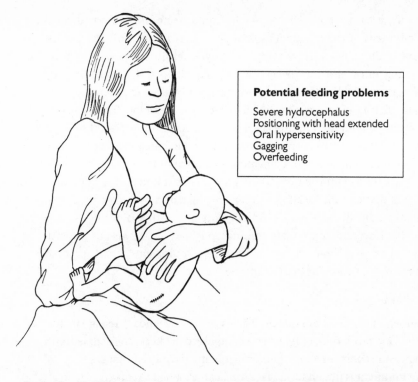

Potential feeding problems

Severe hydrocephalus
Positioning with head extended
Oral hypersensitivity
Gagging
Overfeeding

Figure 5.3. Feeding the baby with spina bifida, and potential feeding problems

Babies with spina bifida may have feeding difficulties because of positioning problems, oral-motor problems, or a combination of both. The newborn baby feeds most easily when the body is totally supported in a semireclined position and her or his head is held slightly forward to facilitate swallowing and prevent choking (Figure 5.3). This may be done while holding the baby or by placing the baby in an infant seat. Positioning problems arise when the infant with spina bifida lacks sufficient head control to maintain the head in the best position for feedings. This may occur because the presence of hydrocephalus makes the head large and difficult to control or because the baby's neck and shoulder girdle muscles are relatively weak. If the baby's head appears to be tilted back or hyperextended during feeding, it may be helpful to place a small pillow or rolled-up towel behind the baby's head (not behind the neck, as this will only increase the hyperextension). Also, the caregiver should avoid being above the eye level of the baby, as this also tends to make the baby hyperextend in an effort to look up.

The process of rooting, suckling, and swallowing is a reflex that comes naturally to newborn babies, yet it requires smooth and coordinated movements of the tongue, lips, and jaw. Many babies with spina bifida have feeding difficulties related to oral hypersensitivity, poor oral-motor control, and a tendency to gag easily. Babies with oral hypersensitivity do not easily tolerate stimulation in or near the mouth. They tend to withdraw, turn away, or fuss when approached with the nipple. They may take the nipple hungrily but quickly reject it, grimace, or gag. Mild findings of oral hypersensitivity are common in babies but are more likely among babies with spina bifida. Feeding problems of this sort are probably caused by the Chiari malformation, which may affect the function of the cranial nerves that control suckling and swallowing. For most babies with such feeding difficulties, patience and diligence are all that is needed to help the baby acquire appropriate feeding skills and to decrease hypersensitivity. For a few babies, however, these feeding problems persist and need more expert treatment (see Chapter 6).

Going Home

Ten years ago, it was common for babies with spina bifida to remain in hospital for many weeks. More recently, improved medical care, coupled with increasing concerns about costs and growing realization that the hospital environment is not an ideal place for a baby, has led to earlier discharges. In the absence of prematurity or some medical complication, it would not be unreasonable for a baby to have the myelomeningocele closed, a shunt placed, sutures removed, and then be ready for discharge home at seven to ten days of age. That places the responsibility on the health care team to ensure that the family is adequately prepared to take care of the baby at home. Preparation prior to discharge from hospital should include the following:

- Teaching the family about spina bifida and ensuring that the caregivers know essential issues related to health care
- Making sure that the parents can manage dressing changes and other aspects of medical care that may be necessary
- Teaching the parents about the signs of hydrocephalus and shunt failure and checking that they can measure head circumference
- Observing feeding closely for evidence of the feeding problems mentioned previously
- Having the parents meet the members of the spina bifida health care team that will be involved in continuing care
- Sharing with the parents information regarding the baby's urological and orthopedic status

- Teaching parents to do appropriate physical therapy interventions, such as range of motion exercises
- Making sure that optimal follow-up is arranged, including community-based primary care and early intervention

Parents and other caregivers should use the time in hospital to get to know the baby and the details of her or his condition. When in doubt, ask questions of the doctors, nurses, and others who are responsible for her or his care. Participate fully in all aspects of daily care, such as feeding, changing, dressing, and the like. Do not let the spina bifida stop you from touching, fondling, and playing with your baby. Gentle handling of this sort is good for your baby and for you too. Your neurosurgeon will give you instructions about the back closure site and the shunt incisions. Generally speaking, the back wound will be well healed before discharge. Although one would avoid pressure over the wound from hard surfaces, common-sense measures are sufficient to prevent damage to the incision. A regular infant car seat should be used for transportation, although I sometimes recommend placing a sanitary pad carefully in the seat to provide more padding and further protection. If your baby has a major spinal deformity, it is a good idea to have a physical therapist or orthotist make a molded insert out of foam to avoid pressure on the skin. Under special circumstances, such as severe kyphosis of the spine, your neurosurgeon may instruct you to avoid having your baby lie completely on his or her back. For most babies, however, this is not a problem. In view of evidence that lying face down may increase the risk of sudden infant death syndrome (SIDS), lying on the side with a small towel roll for support may work well.

Thinking about the Future

Leaving the hospital is the end of one important chapter in the life of your new baby but also the beginning of a much greater saga. This can be an exhausting time of anxiety, demoralization, and sleepless nights. It is also a time when your mind turns to the future. What will she be? What will life be like for her as she grows up with a physical disability? How will this affect her? How will we deal with whatever may be in store? These are unanswerable questions, but it is vital that you think about them or share your worries and fears with another person. These realistic concerns for the future will help you to be prepared, to make good decisions, and to foster a family environment that will encourage your child to adapt and to cope with adversity.

MEDICAL ISSUES

Closure of Open Myelomeningoceles

There are three important reasons for closing an open myelomeningocele. The first and most urgent reason is to prevent infection. The open neural placode is quickly colonized with bacteria after birth, and the bacteria can easily infect the CSF, causing meningitis. The second reason is to preserve existing nerve function, which requires meticulous care of the sac before surgery and special operative techniques during surgery. The third reason to close the defect is to minimize later orthopedic deformities of the spine (kyphoscoliosis).

After delivery, the myelomeningocele should be protected from further injury and potential infection. If the myelomeningocele sac is intact and full of fluid, special efforts should be taken to avoid rupture. Once the baby is stable, the following steps are taken:

1. The sac is covered loosely with a warm, sterile dressing.
2. The dressing is kept moist with saline.
3. An IV (intravenous line) is started to give antibiotics.
4. Handling of the baby is minimized (although there should always be the opportunity for early cuddling if the baby's condition is stable).
5. The baby should be positioned prone or on his or her side.
6. Plans are made for the neurosurgeon to close the back.

As a general rule, the back should be closed within forty-eight hours of birth and preferably within twenty-four hours. This gives enough time to ensure that the baby is stable and in optimal medical condition before surgery. It also provides sufficient time to investigate the degree of hydrocephalus, to examine the baby carefully for the existence of any other problems or congenital abnormalities, and to plan the optimal surgical approach to achieve closure. It affords a window for some quiet time for the parent(s) to be with the baby and for the process of bonding to be facilitated. Under some circumstances, difficult decisions regarding treatment options may necessitate delaying closure of the myelomeningocele for a few days. Although controversial, it may be possible to wait for five or six days without increasing the chances of serious infections or tethering.

The neurosurgeon bases the decision regarding the best method of closure on the size of the sac, its position on the back, and the presence of associated bone abnormalities of the spine. There are three aspects to closure that must be considered: (1) the closure of the neural elements, (2) the surrounding bone and muscle tissue, and (3) the skin.

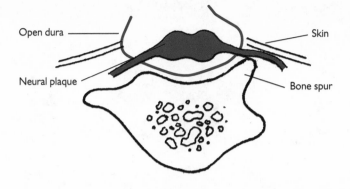

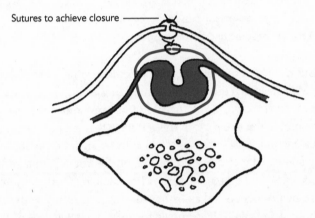

Figure 5.4. Closure of an open myelomeningocele. The neurosurgeon must carefully dissect the neural plaque, trim any troublesome bone spurs, and take care to achieve a watertight closure of the dura.

First, the neural elements themselves must be meticulously dissected. The neural placode needs to be carefully inspected, and any tethering bands and bone spurs that may cause subsequent problems should be removed. Next, the neural placode needs to be closed and covered by watertight closure of the dura (Figure 5.4). Some neurosurgeons attempt to reconstitute the tubular configuration of the normal spinal cord by rolling up the neural placode, whereas others routinely replace the neural placode into the spinal canal without first doing so-called entubulation. In all cases, the dura must be tightly closed over the neural placode to prevent leaks.

One of the complications of closure is the development of severe

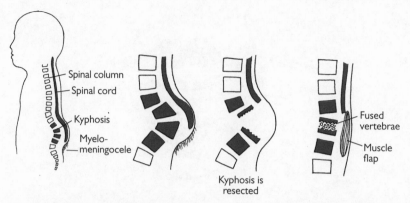

Figure 5.5. Surgical treatment of severe kyphosis associated with a myelomeningocele. It is sometimes necessary to remove parts of the vertebrae to produce a straighter spine and better closure.

kyphoscoliosis and other spinal orthopedic deformities. The neurosurgeon therefore needs to consider the surrounding bone and muscle tissue. If there is a severe kyphosis at the site of the myelomeningocele, it is usually helpful to remove parts of the vertebrae that are jutting out from the rest of the spine at the time of initial closure (Figure 5.5). This procedure may allow better closure and healing of the wound. Some of these operations can be quite extensive, lasting hours and requiring the joint expertise of a neurosurgeon and an orthopedic surgeon. Other spurs of protruding bone may need to be trimmed to create a relatively even surface at the site of closure, thereby preventing later pressure areas and potential sites of wound breakdown. Often, strips of muscle are placed over the dural closure to add further protection and to help prevent leaks.

Finally, the neurosurgeon must consider the most suitable kind of skin closure. The kinds of closure are shown in Figure 5.6. When possible, a primary longitudinal closure in the midline is preferred for small lesions. Generally, myelomeningoceles that are associated with a skin defect less than half the width of the back can be closed directly by this method. Larger lesions typically need an oval-shaped skin graft or a graft with lateral relaxing incisions. Following the closure, care is taken to avoid pressure over the site of closure until the wound is well healed, usually around one to two weeks, although this may take longer if the closure was a difficult procedure.

Hydrocephalus

It is important to assess the presence and degree of hydrocephalus of newborn babies with spina bifida. Not every baby with spina bifida develops

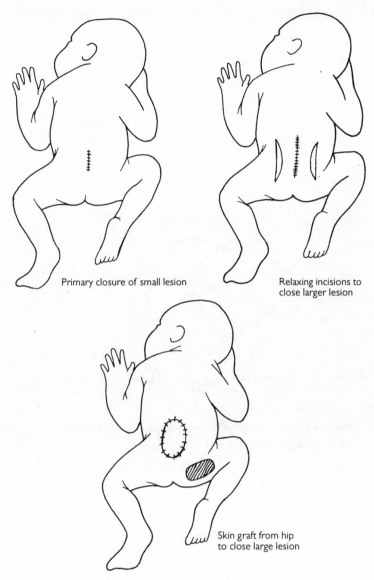

Primary closure of small lesion

Relaxing incisions to close larger lesion

Skin graft from hip to close large lesion

Figure 5.6. Different methods of skin closure: larger lesions usually need relaxing incisions and/or skin grafts.

hydrocephalus. Indeed, about 5–10 percent of babies (and almost 20 percent of those with small, sacral-level lesions) do not require a shunt. There are many signs of hydrocephalus in the newborn on clinical examination (Figure 5.7). In many cases the hydrocephalus is immediately obvious. The baby may have a large head circumference because the soft, malleable skull of the newborn is pushed outward by the enlarging CSF spaces.

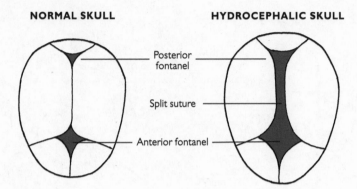

NORMAL SKULL   HYDROCEPHALIC SKULL

Posterior fontanel

Split suture

Anterior fontanel

SPLIT SUTURE

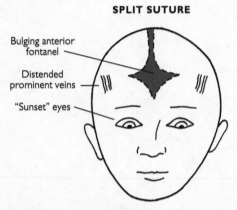

Bulging anterior fontanel

Distended prominent veins

"Sunset" eyes

Figure 5.7. Hydrocephalus in the newborn. Large head circumference, wide open and full fontanels, and split sutures indicate enlarging CSF spaces. Other clinical signs include distended veins and a "sunset" appearance to the eyes.

The anterior and posterior fontanels are enlarged and have an unmistakable fullness to the gentle touch. The midline suture may be split wide apart, which the examiner can appreciate by running a finger back in the midline from the anterior fontanel. However, more subtle cases of hydrocephalus may not be clearly evident to the clinician. In all newborns with spina bifida, it is therefore essential to obtain a computerized tomography (CT) scan or head ultrasound scan.

Head ultrasound scans can be easily accomplished by holding a probe at the anterior fontanel (the "soft spot," which is wide open in babies) and have the advantage of not involving X-rays. For babies who are not medically stable, such a scan may be done at the bedside in the nursery.

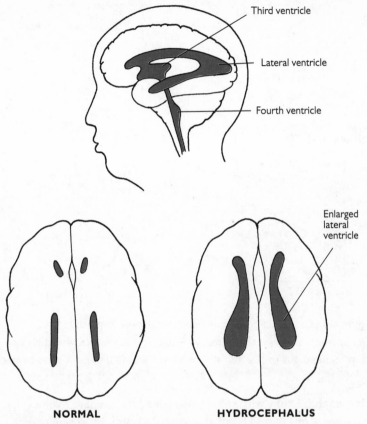

Figure 5.8. Typical appearances of a CT scan in a newborn with hydrocephalus. Notice the enlarged lateral ventricles.

Head CT scans are also easily obtained and do not require administration of any sedation or intravenous dye. Typical appearances of neonatal head CT scans are shown in Figure 5.8.

The scans are vital for the neurosurgeon to decide whether a shunt is needed and whether any other visible abnormalities of the brain may need monitoring. If the scan indicates minimal or no hydrocephalus, the neurosurgeon may decide to monitor the baby's head closely, which may include measuring head circumference each day and plotting the measurements on a chart at the bedside, as well as routinely repeating the ultrasound scan if there is clinical evidence of progressive hydrocephalus. Not infrequently, CSF pressure changes that occur following back closure lead to progressive hydrocephalus, requiring placement of a shunt (Figure 5.9). Although hydrocephalus can develop at any time, it is gener-

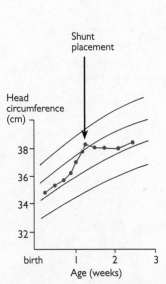

Head circumference

Measure at widest part
Measure twice
Record longer
  measurement
Record carefully

Figure 5.9. Careful daily measurements of the newborn baby's head circumference may reveal progressive hydrocephalus, which would require the placement of a shunt. Also shown are the essential steps in measurement.

ally true that a baby with spina bifida who does not have hydrocephalus at the age of one month is unlikely to need a shunting procedure later.

Shunt Procedures

Neurosurgeons have long struggled with the problems of treating hydrocephalus in children. Research in the earlier part of this century clarified the mechanisms of CSF production, absorption, pressure, and flow, leading to the development of surgical operations to shunt and drain CSF. However, these early shunt procedures frequently contributed to erosion of tissues, toxic effects on the brain, obstructions, infections, or death. Over the past thirty years, a number of important advances and technical innovations have improved the success rates of shunting from less than 50 percent to over 90 percent. Among these advances is the dramatic contribution of engineer Dr. John Holter.

In 1956, Holter's only son, Casey, was born with a myelomeningocele. He recovered from an early bout of meningitis and then developed hydrocephalus. Two attempts were made at placing a shunt of polyethylene tubing, but these were unsuccessful. The baby's father used his engineering skills to develop a dual-valve system with a new material called Silastic. Dr. G. Spitz, a resident in neurosurgery at the Children's Hospital of Philadelphia, agreed to insert the new ventriculo-atrial shunt. The shunt worked well for fourteen months before it became occluded. Casey's father again worked closely with Spitz to develop a revised shunt system, which again worked well until Casey died of intractable seizures at the age of five. Holter continued to work tirelessly on perfecting shunt valves. He formed an independent company, and during the following twenty years, he and his colleagues made many significant advances that have revolutionized the treatment of hydrocephalus.

Since the early innovations of Dr. Holter, a number of other refinements have been made to improve the functioning of shunts. Small reservoirs have been added to allow access to the CSF for evaluation or treatment of infection. Chambers with valves give doctors opportunities to assess filling and emptying of reservoirs, which can be useful in determining whether a shunt is blocked or not functioning properly. Valves allow drainage of CSF above certain threshold pressures, thereby preventing sudden, excessive decompression of the ventricles. Newer materials are used for shunt tubing to prevent kinking or damage to body tissues or organs and to enable the tubing to show up well on X-rays. There are many shunt systems available, and different neurosurgeons have different preferences. Most often, newborns with spina bifida and hydrocephalus are given a Holter, Hakim, or Pudenz-Schultz system (Figure 5.10).

Shunts can drain CSF into several locations, including the peritoneal space (the abdominal cavity), atrium (the small chamber of the heart), the gallbladder, or directly to the outside of the head (external ventricular drainage). In almost all cases, newborns have a ventriculo-peritoneal shunt placed so that the CSF drains into the space surrounding the abdominal organs, as this arrangement has been shown to have fewer complications than does ventriculo-atrial shunting.

The routine newborn shunt procedure takes about ninety minutes and is done under general anesthesia. Part of the scalp is shaved and an incision is made on one side of the head. The ventricular catheter is guided through a small hole in the skull into the frontal part of the ventricle on one side. Since the ventricles are connected, there is generally no reason to have more than one ventricular catheter. The position of the shunt is checked and then fixed. The reservoir system is attached and put in place. The distal end is placed into the abdomen after tunneling the tubing under the skin. Antibiotics are generally given around the time of surgery to help prevent infection of the shunt.

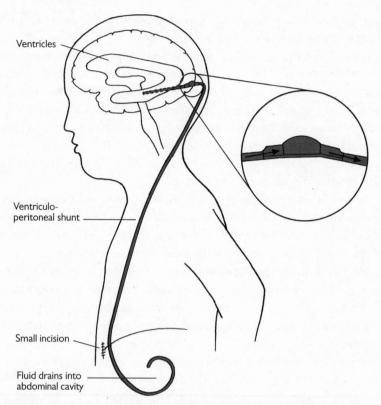

Ventricles

Ventriculo-
peritoneal shunt

Small incision

Fluid drains into
abdominal cavity

Figure 5.10. The appearance and mechanism of a ventriculo-peritoneal shunt system. Excess CSF drains from the ventricles through the ventricular catheter, shunt valve, and shunt tubing into the abdominal cavity.

Following the surgery, care is taken to protect the wound. A dressing is applied, after which the neurosurgeons and nursing staff check the wound daily. Head ultrasound or CT scans may be used to determine the extent to which the ventricle size decreases. Also, the head circumference and clinical examination of the baby's head can provide valuable information.

Ideally, the shunt should allow controlled drainage, so that the rate of head growth is normal. This usually means that the ventricles continue to look a little enlarged on follow-up scans. The shunting is not expected to take away the hydrocephalus completely but to prevent progressive hydrocephalus. Mild to moderate hydrocephalus or ventricular enlargement may persist; what matters is whether this degree of hydrocephalus changes on further follow-up. The so-called slit ventricle syndrome may result if the shunt decompresses the ventricles excessively or at very low pressure. If the shunt functions only at very high pressure, progressive hydrocephalus may occur. New shunt systems have been designed to respond to a range of pressure changes, such as postural changes, coughing, and physical exertion, automatically varying shunt resistance to regulate the rate of drainage. There are even shunts that are electronically programmable, like pacemakers, so that they can be adjusted to deal with different circumstances. Shunts will be discussed further in the section on shunt failure in the next chapter.

Chiari Malformation

One hundred years ago, Professor H. Chiari, a German pathologist, observed a malformation of the brain that was present in a group of patients. The essential feature of the Chiari malformation is the downward displacement of a portion of the brain into the neck, occurring in three distinct levels of severity, from Type I (the mildest form) to Type III (the most severe). Individuals with spina bifida have the intermediate form of Chiari malformation (Type II), and this malformation is present to some degree in almost all patients.

Although the most obvious aspect of the Chiari II malformation is in the cerebellum and brainstem, the malformation is pancephalic—that is, it is accompanied by anatomic differences in other parts of the brain as well. A discussion of the embryonic development of this malformation is included in Chapter 2. Figure 5.11 shows some of the features of the malformation, including the downward displacement of the cerebellar vermis, the elongation of the medulla and the fourth ventricle, and the kinking of the medulla over the cervical spinal cord.

The Chiari II malformation may present symptoms at any age and is therefore an important topic to which we will return when we discuss medical issues for toddlers (Chapter 6) and adolescents (Chapter 9). Whereas "brain in the neck" commonly causes pain in the neck in older children, infants may face the life-threatening Chiari crisis. The Chiari crisis of infancy is related to brainstem and lower cranial nerve dysfunction. Affected babies usually manifest a weak or absent cry and stridor (obstructed or high-pitched sounds on breathing in). For some, the respiratory symptoms are so acute that the infants stop breathing for prolonged periods (apnea), drop their heart rates, and become dusky blue (cyanosis). Many have severe feeding and swallowing disorders, with extreme arching of the neck, gastroesophageal reflux, and failure to thrive. Approximately one in three babies with spina bifida have mild symptoms of the Chiari II malformation, including the feeding difficulties that were

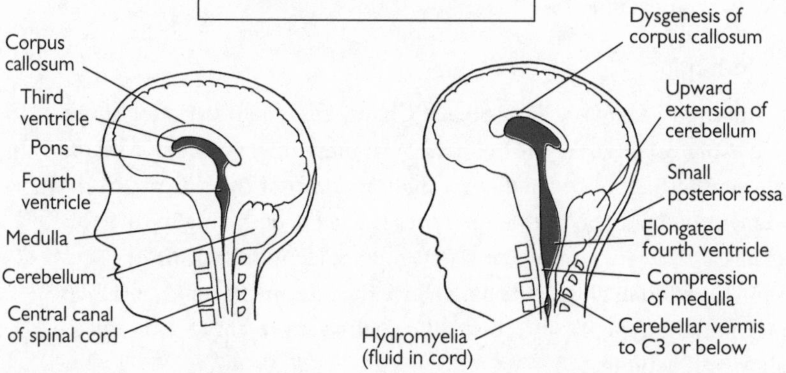

Figure 5.11. Features of the Chiari II malformation, compared with normal anatomy (left), as shown on an MRI scan. Notice the poorly formed corpus callosum and the downward displacement of the cerebellum, which may lead to brainstem compression symptoms, as given in the box.

mentioned earlier in the chapter. A much smaller proportion, around one in twenty, have the more severe symptoms of brainstem dysfunction described above.

There appears to be a spectrum of involvement of the brainstem. Milder symptoms may be related to traction on the lower cranial nerves and compression of the brainstem. More severe symptoms may be associated with actual hemorrhages or areas of infarction in the brainstem. If these areas correspond to vital structures and cranial nerve nuclei, they may be evident as an absent gag reflex, altered respiratory drive, and abnormal carbon dioxide (CO_2) response curves.

Assessment of the Chiari II malformation requires an MRI scan to visualize clearly the hindbrain and spinal cord. If the junction between brainstem and spinal cord is at the level of C4 or below, the likelihood of significant Chiari symptoms is high. It is also essential to determine whether the shunt is working properly. The role of such other tests as the CO_2 response test, somatosensory-evoked potentials, and brainstem auditory–evoked poten-

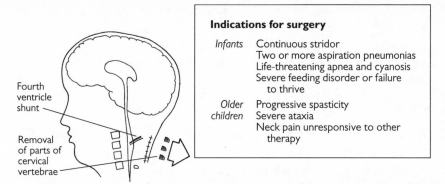

Indications for surgery

Infants	Continuous stridor
	Two or more aspiration pneumonias
	Life-threatening apnea and cyanosis
	Severe feeding disorder or failure to thrive
Older children	Progressive spasticity
	Severe ataxia
	Neck pain unresponsive to other therapy

Fourth ventricle shunt

Removal of parts of cervical vertebrae

Figure 5.12. Surgical management of the Chiari II malformation and indications for surgery, which usually entails the removal of part of the cervical vertebrae and/or the placement of a shunt at the fourth ventricle

tials has not been clearly defined, but these tests may provide reassuring evidence of the basic integrity of the brainstem.

The most disconcerting aspect of the treatment of the Chiari crisis of infancy is the unpredictability of outcomes. Of those with clear evidence of central ventilatory dysfunction, almost 50 percent die in spite of aggressive treatment. Babies who manifest only stridor have a better prognosis. Many improve spontaneously, with symptoms gradually resolving within one to two years. Such infants may have clear evidence of laryngeal dysfunction on bronchoscopy and may be prone to aspiration and reflux. Some will have vocal cord paralysis and may even need tracheostomy for prolonged periods. Careful attention to feeding, nutrition, respiratory function, and adequacy of shunt function is essential while waiting for the baby to outgrow the Chiari II symptoms. Parents need to be trained in the use of home monitors, tracheostomy care, and resuscitation. Such home-based vigilance is extremely demanding for parents and must be coupled with extensive support.

For those babies with progressive, life-threatening symptoms, surgery may be curative. Indications for surgery are shown in Figure 5.12. The options include decompressing the brainstem by removing the back of the cervical vertebrae and the lowest part of the skull and/or the placement of a shunt at the fourth ventricle. The former procedure serves to unroof the cervical spine, thereby relieving pressure on the low-lying brainstem. The surgery is technically difficult and requires an experienced neurosurgeon. Unfortunately, those with severe symptoms may fail to improve or may have short-lived improvement in brainstem function. In these circumstances, repeat operations are not beneficial. It appears that some Chiari II malformations in infants are beyond repair and that it may be advantageous to operate early on the small minority of severely symptomatic babies.

Ventriculitis

In the past, many newborn babies underwent closure and shunting, only to develop bacterial infections of the shunt, meninges, and ventricles (ventriculitis). Major intracranial infections of this kind were often devastating in their effects. Many babies succumbed in spite of antibiotics, and most of the survivors were neurologically impaired. Almost all the severely retarded children whom I see in clinic had this problem in infancy. There are two children, now in their late teens, who developed severe shunt infections and ventriculitis as infants. Prolonged efforts to treat their infections were unsuccessful, and when the doctors eventually felt that there was nothing more to offer, their parents requested that they take the babies home. The doctors agreed, anticipating that they would soon die. Contrary to expectations, the babies were gradually nursed back to health. Unfortunately, however, their developmental outcomes have been very poor. Complications of this kind were not rare. In one large series (Lorber 1972), 18 percent of the babies developed ventriculitis as newborns. By contrast, only 2.5 percent of a more recent series (McLone et al. 1982) developed this complication. The improvement probably reflects improved surgical techniques, advances in medical care of the newborn baby, and more effective antibiotics.

If a recently shunted baby develops a fever, vomiting, seizures, or other signs of infection, it is essential to obtain cultures from the blood, urine, and, most important, from the shunt itself. The baby should be started on broad-spectrum antibiotics (such as vancomycin and cefotaxime) while awaiting the results of the investigations. If there are indications of shunt infection, most neurosurgeons will remove the existing shunt and, if CSF drainage is needed, place a new shunt that drains into a sterile system outside the baby (external ventricular drainage). The fluid can be accessed periodically to ensure that it is clearing in response to the treatment. Antibiotics are administered intravenously; under some circumstances, the antibiotics can be administered safely into the ventricles in order to provide more potent activity against the infecting bacteria. The duration of antibiotic therapy in cases of ventriculitis is typically around two to three weeks. The neurosurgeon usually replaces a ventriculo-peritoneal shunt at the completion of the antibiotic course. The outlook these days for ventriculitis that is diagnosed quickly and treated aggressively is excellent. In fact, one of the smartest toddlers in our clinic is a little fellow who spent the first six weeks in hospital with a severe E. coli ventriculitis!

Urodynamics and the "Hostile Bladder"

Urinary tract problems in the newborn period are not very common. However, the potential cost of missing a condition that is easily treatable and threatens to damage the infant's kidneys is enormous. Ninety percent of newborns with spina bifida have normal urinary tracts on ultrasound examination at birth. These scans provide very clear images of the kidneys and ureters (upper urinary tracts) and the bladder. A few will be found to have congenital anomalies of the kidneys, such as horseshoe kidney, that are of little clinical significance. Unfortunately, by the age of five, some children will have developed worrisome changes in their kidneys, such as hydronephrosis and renal scarring. How does this happen, and what can be done to prevent it? The challenge is to detect and provide early treatment for those babies who have a so-called hostile bladder and who are at risk of upper-tract deterioration.

Urodynamics (also known as Video Uro-Dynamic Studies, or VUDS) is a valuable tool for diagnosing and monitoring the hostile bladder. The technique involves a fairly elaborate recording of bladder pressure and volume (also known as a cystometrogram, or CMG) as well as a recording of muscle activity from the bladder neck (an electromyogram, or EMG), all done under visual control using low X-ray exposure. If we were to do urodynamics on all newborns with spina bifida (as is practiced routinely in many centers where urodynamic studies are readily available), we would find that about one-third had high bladder pressures and a bladder outlet muscle that did not relax appropriately. This latter finding goes by the awkward name of detrusor-sphincter dyssynergia, or DSD (Figure 5.13). If we were to follow a group of untreated babies with high pressures and DSD, we would find that almost half of them developed hydronephrosis over time. This occurs because high pressures generated in the bladder as it contracts against a tight sphincter are transmitted up the ureters and cause them to weaken and balloon out at the level of the kidneys. It is for this reason that the hostile bladder needs treatment. Fortunately, the use of clean intermittent catheterization (CIC), which we will discuss in depth in Chapter 8, and anticholinergic medication substantially decreases the bladder pressures. In one series, only two of twenty-six infants with hostile bladders who were treated with CIC and anticholinergics went on to

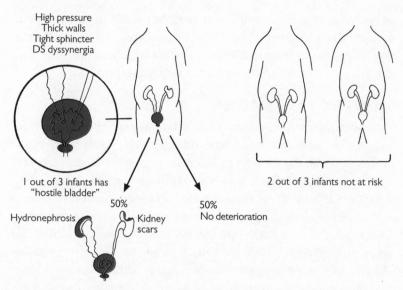

High pressure
Thick walls
Tight sphincter
DS dyssynergia

I out of 3 infants has
"hostile bladder"

Hydronephrosis

50%

Kidney
scars

50%
No deterioration

2 out of 3 infants not at risk

Figure 5.13. The "hostile bladder" and its potential effects on the kidneys if left untreated. Appropriate treatment can prevent hydronephrosis and kidney scars.

develop hydronephrosis. Such treatment is clearly the standard of care for newborns with a hostile bladder. If CIC is not a practical solution or is ineffective, vesicostomy, a relatively simple operation to drain the bladder and prevent high bladder pressure, is an effective short-term solution.

Many urologists recommend obtaining urodynamics in all newborns with spina bifida and assessing the degree of hostility. Those with high "hostility scores" are treated and then followed very closely for evidence of upper-tract changes. The evidence suggests that almost 40 percent of those infants with high scores develop upper-tract changes, compared with only around 10 percent of those with low scores. However, urodynamic studies are expensive, invasive, and not readily available in all centers. It is not clear that all babies need this kind of initial evaluation. First, there is a very easy test that may pick up most of the babies with DSD quite effectively. Babies with DSD would be expected to have incomplete emptying of their bladders, so that large, postvoid residual urine volumes would suggest the presence of DSD. It is a good idea to perform a few catheterizations immediately after urination is observed in the newborn period and record the amount of urine in the bladder. Postvoid residual volumes of 20 cc or more suggest DSD. Second, babies with DSD tend to get bacteria colonizing or infecting their bladders; thus the finding of bacteria on a screening urine examination should raise suspicions of a hostile bladder. Third, it is frequently observed that mild hydronephrosis in infancy is reversible, so that the institution of CIC and anticholinergics after the appearance of hydronephrosis on routine ultrasound is usually effective in treating the problem. For these reasons, an acceptable alternative to routine urodynamics on all newborns may be screening every three months with examinations of postvoid residuals and catheterized urine samples, as well as renal ultrasound examinations every four to six months during the first year. Those babies with upper-tract changes of hydronephrosis or hydroureter and those with bacteriuria or high postvoid residuals should be referred for urodynamics. A high index of suspicion for the hostile bladder and a readiness to treat with CIC and anticholinergics is recommended to prevent kidney damage.

Vesico-Ureteral Reflux

Another urinary tract condition that occurs quite commonly in the child with spina bifida is reflux of urine from the bladder up into the ureters (vesico-ureteral reflux), which should not be confused with gastroesophageal reflux, in which babies spit up excessively. Vesico-ureteral reflux may occur in association with high bladder pressures. Because this problem is more likely to arise later in childhood, I will return to this subject in Chapter 8. It is worth mentioning here that about 5 percent of newborns with spina bifida have reflux, but this is usually mild and tends to resolve itself over time if bladder function is adequate. Babies with reflux should be on prophylactic antibiotics to prevent infections, since bladder infections are more likely to damage the kidneys if the infected urine is refluxing up the ureters. It is also better to avoid doing crede (massaging the lower abdomen to stimulate complete emptying of the bladder) in babies with reflux. Most babies with reflux can be effectively managed with CIC, which results in complete resolution in about two-thirds of the children.

Sometimes, however, surgery is indicated in early infancy to treat reflux. Usually this involves reimplantation of the ureters into the bladder in such a way as to prevent reflux. Reimplantation is frequently combined with augmentation of the bladder, a surgical procedure in which a segment of bowel is attached to the bladder to enlarge its capacity. Bladder augmentation procedures are discussed in Chapter 8 in the section on surgical management of incontinence.

ETHICAL ISSUES

A complete discussion of the ethical issues that may arise in the care of newborns with spina bifida is beyond the scope of this book. A few specific circumstances may arise, however, in which parents and doctors have to confront agonizing ethical decisions. It is helpful to place the current situation in a historical context.

In the late 1960s and early 1970s, most centers practiced nonselective treatment of babies with spina bifida. In other words, nearly all babies were treated with closure of the spine. In 1971, Dr. J. Lorber published a very large retrospective series of 524 unselected cases and, through a process of thorough description of the outcomes of these cases, proposed that the presence of certain adverse features at birth spelled a poor outcome. From this and other work grew the practice of selective treatment of newborns, so that babies with thoracic lesions, severe hydrocephalus, and other congenital anomalies were frequently not operated on and were given supportive treatment to keep them comfortable until they died. This is still the case in many parts of the world. In the United States, the days of selective treatment of babies with spina bifida are over. The turning point occurred in 1983, when the Reagan administration published regulations (the Baby Doe regulations) under which no infant, by virtue of spina bifida or other birth defect, could be denied therapy. Although there have been no cases brought successfully against doctors, these regulations significantly changed the practice of pediatrics. No longer was it permissible for doctors to "play God" in the nursery by making decisions based on quality of life. Instead, there developed a greater sensitivity to parents' emotional needs and to the need for consensus among caregivers. Ethics committees were established in hospitals and procedures worked out for obtaining valuable guidance from such committees when ethical questions arose.

When making proxy decisions on behalf of infants, we always struggle to determine what is "in the child's best interests." The age-old ethical questions surrounding the sanctity of life versus the quality of life are immensely difficult ones. Some might argue that decisions about selection and nontreatment are moral questions and are therefore not the business of doctors, parents, or anyone else but the courts. I cannot agree with this position: the suspension of judgment and its replacement with fear of litigation or prosecution is no solution.

In my opinion, there are compelling arguments, both ethical and medical, against selection. First, the poor predictability of outcomes argues strongly against selective treatment. I have seen many babies with severe hydrocephalus in utero and at birth whose later development was similar to others with minimal or mild hydrocephalus. I have also seen a baby with multiple congenital anomalies and severe scoliosis in addition to thoracic spina bifida, one whom many of us might have considered for nontreatment; indeed, had his parents indicated a wish not to proceed with closure, we would almost certainly have discussed it with our ethics committee and gone along with the parents' wishes. In this case, his parents were adamant about doing all that could be done, and now, four years later, he is doing better than I or any of the health care team expected.

Second, those of us who staff clinics for children with spina bifida know of children who were selected for nontreatment, who were supposed to die, but who survived in spite of all odds. It is likely that the quality of life for such unexpected survivors is poorer than it would otherwise have been had they been offered full treatment as newborns.

Although many people were reviled by Lorber's cold, logical analysis and its implications, his work certainly made physicians take stock of the situation twenty years ago and consider their role in ethical decision making. I believe that the physician's role in ethical decision making in the 1990s is to inform and advise parents about likely outcomes, acknowledging that there is a huge amount of uncertainty. Parents, on the other hand, have to live with their decisions. Major treatment decisions such as these seldom rest on objective criteria, instead depending on the parents' individual experiences, values, and subjective feelings. They need to be involved at every step.

PARENT-TO-PARENT

"When Julia was born, I felt totally confused, almost paralyzed. I couldn't even think straight. It all seemed totally overwhelming, and every minute of every day and night there was nothing there but her spina bifida and the deepest grief I had ever known.

And then, gradually, I began to notice other things. Her mouth, her fingers—little things like that. And that feeling of helplessness began to pass."

"When Chris was born, it was a surprise to myself, my husband, and the medical staff to see a large, open myelomeningocele on the back of this robust baby! As information came to us about spina bifida and hydrocephalus, in our fear and sense of insecurity we instinctively turned to prayer. I secretly prayed that God would take my son to Heaven, partly because I didn't want him to suffer and partly to take away my own pain and feelings of inadequacy. As time went on I came to realize that God does work miracles these days. Most of all I realized that God often uses people, like doctors, other parents, and family, to bring those miracles into our world."

Infants and Toddlers

I n our clinics, we like to organize our appointments by age group, thus seeing children of similar ages on any given day. One week we may see children of school age, the next week mainly older adolescents and young adults, and so on. Although each of these age groups has its specific charm, no group warms the heart like the infants and toddlers! These kids are growing and developing before our very eyes and are a continual source of gratification and wonder to their parents. The members of our clinic team take great delight in sharing in the care of the infants and toddlers, partly, I think, because we see so much potential in these little kids and feel optimistic in our efforts to help them to realize that potential. I hope that this optimism and clear sense of purpose is evident in this chapter.

Chapter 6 is concerned with the age range of approximately six to thirty-six months. It begins with an overview of the important areas of development in this age range and the ways in which early intervention at home by parents and therapists can facilitate such development. The benefits of early walking and the methods of achieving upright posture are discussed in depth. Other topics important for the habilitation and medical needs of this age group are also included.

DEVELOPMENTAL ISSUES

Progressions and Expectations

Benjamin Spock wrote of "the passion to explore" that characterizes the behavior of a one-year-old child. How to deal effectively with a wandering baby and make his environment safe is a perennial problem for parents of infants and toddlers. Erik Erikson, the great psychoanalyst, wrote eloquently about the other essential developmental characteristic of this age group—namely, the drive toward autonomy. He described how the matu-

Aspects of development	Six months	Twelve months
Adaptive	Visually directed grasp	Voluntary release of objects Feeds self cracker, Cheerios May reach across midline
Fine-motor	Raking grasp Emerging hand-to-hand transfer	Mature pincer grasp Transfers easily from hand to hand Holds cup
Gross-motor	Rolls over Sits with support	May throw objects Crawling, creeping Pulling to stand
Language	Vocalizes, babbling Reciprocal vocalization	Imitates sounds First words Pointing at objects Follows one-step commands
Cognitive	Persists in playing with toy for longer period	Object permanence mastered Active experimentation with toys
Personal-social	Laughs out loud Shows delight with parent contact	Loves to play peek-a-boo Shows stranger anxiety

Figure 6.1. Developmental milestones in children from six to thirty-six months, showing anticipated changes in adaptive, fine-motor, gross-motor, language, cognitive, and personal-social skills

ration of the motor system allows the infant to drop and throw things at will, by which "the still highly dependent child begins to endow his autonomous will." These struggles of autonomy are evident in the infant who refuses his food, in the temper tantrums of the toddler, and in the small child who won't stay in bed at night. The coordination of conflicting patterns of "holding on" and "letting go" are also played out in the arena of toilet training, as a toddler learns to evacuate bowel and bladder voluntarily, to the cheers and delight of parents!

What are the implications, then, for infants and toddlers with spina bifida, whose neurologic condition affects motor coordination, independent mobility, and control of bowel and bladder? Are the drives to explore the environment and to exercise autonomous will absent or different? Fortunately, the answer is a resounding "No"! Babies with spina bifida are also motivated to master their environments, and toddlers with spina bifida may show an awareness and interest in toileting and a readiness to gain control of these processes. Even when certain muscle groups do not

Twenty-four months	Thirty-six months
Uses spoon Drinks from cup without spilling	Uses fork
Increasing dexterity	Handedness usually emerging
Walking	Improving balance Postural control and coordination
Puts two words together Dramatic increase in vocabulary	Speaks in short sentences Use of pronouns Understands prepositions Identifies body parts Speech mostly intelligible
Emerging pretend play	Scribbles with pencil Copies circle
Less anxious Explores new environments Attaches to transitional objects Parallel play	Ventures out Socializes with strangers Cooperative social play

work and when mobility is impaired, the drive toward exploration is still present in infancy. If opportunities to learn through exploration are limited, however, that internal motivation may tend to become blunted. By way of compensation, some infants and toddlers will become very skilled at engaging the assistance of adults to get their needs met. The strategy becomes, "If I can't do it myself, I suppose I'll get somebody to help." To some extent, the challenge for the parent changes from one of controlling the environment and making it safe to one of *introducing* the environment and making it *accessible*, thereby encouraging self-reliance.

One useful way of teasing apart and understanding the complex phenomena of early child development is to consider separate but interrelated streams of development. I like to consider six different aspects of development which are discernible in infancy and which can be followed through early childhood and on into school-age children. They are (1) adaptive behavior, (2) gross-motor development, (3) fine-motor development, (4) language development, (5) cognitive development, and (6) personal-social development (Figure 6.1). These streams of development can be assessed by various techniques at different ages. Certain aspects of development may strongly affect certain other aspects. For example, toddlers with language delays may have problems in the personal-social domain. The different streams of development may be dissociated, however, so that it is not uncommon for infants and toddlers to show strengths in certain areas and weaknesses in others. Moreover, there tends to be continuity along these developmental streams; therefore a given profile of strengths and weaknesses is commonly maintained as a child becomes older. I have often seen infants with spina bifida who are particularly verbal and social and show significant fine-motor delay and who continue to demonstrate this pattern of strengths and weaknesses by the time they reach kindergarten.

Adaptive behavior refers to the infant's resourcefulness, problem solving, and organization. It includes the way an infant coordinates eyes and hands in reaching for and manipulating a toy, the ability to make adjustments or utilize materials to attain a goal, and the process of learning from experience to solve new problems. It is related to our concepts of intelligence, and it undoubtedly is assisted by (among other things) attention, memory, and a facilitating environment that is rich in experience.

Gross-motor development includes head control, postural reactions, and control of the large muscles of the trunk and limbs. It is the system that underlies the orderly and sequential development of mobility, from rolling to independent sitting, creeping, crawling, and walking. Gross-motor development tends to progress "from head to tail," starting with head control and proceeding to the trunk, arms, and legs. It also tends to proceed from the proximal parts of limbs (nearer the trunk) to the distal parts (nearer the hands and feet). Gross-motor development is intimately connected with the sensory system, in that movement is regulated by the integration of a variety of senses—for example, touch (sensation), vision (spatial awareness), and balance (vestibular system).

Fine-motor development consists of the use of hands and fingers to grasp and manipulate toys and objects. Infants progress from a relatively unrefined raking of objects (six months) to an immature grasp involving thumb and side of the forefinger (inferior scissors grasp, eight months) before developing a more mature pincer grasp (ten months). Fine-motor development is also related to spatial awareness and sensory integration, in that these sensory systems facilitate the ability of infants to plan a sequence of movements (motor planning).

Language development includes all forms of communication, including the use of gesture, facial expressions, and preverbal vocalizations that are communicative in nature. Smiling and cooing are among the earlier forms of communication. Subsequently, more complex sounds are imitated, followed by words, and then combinations of words, which are learned from and reinforced by parents and others. The sequence of language development is orderly and predictable.

Cognitive development refers to the infant's capacity to learn, to remember, and to master a range of skills. These thinking and problem-solving skills are critical in the development of academic achievement and creativity.

Personal-social development refers to the extent to which the toddler is meeting developmentally appropriate social expectations. It includes the child's self-help skills, such as feeding, dressing, and toileting. It also includes the child's independent play skills and the readiness to show cooperation and positive social behavior in groups.

Exploration and Experience

The things children learn about their environment clearly form the basis of subsequent learning. Parents can help their infants and toddlers with spina bifida experience different environments in several ways. First, and most important, remember that infants need to explore with their mouths. Early hand-to-mouth activities and mouthing of toys are critical for the development of later self-feeding skills. It is helpful to place a young infant's hands on the bottle or breast during feeding. Encouraging finger feeding and food play at around seven to eight months of age is an enjoyable activity, and mess should be tolerated if not actually encouraged! Your infant should be helped to hold a bottle and encouraged to do so independently by around eight to eleven months. The cup can be introduced at about twelve to fifteen months of age, as well as self-feeding with a spoon. Spills and other hazards can be decreased (but not totally eliminated) by using a weighted cup, a scoop dish with steep sides, and a nonslip place mat. Of course, many children with spina bifida lack the motor coordination to do some of these skills at the usual time, and some have feeding problems related to the Chiari malformation. Some specific strategies for the management of Chiari-related, oral-motor feeding problems are discussed later in the chapter.

Second, infants love to explore different textures of play materials. Stock the playroom with a variety of toys, including things that are soft and furry and rough and coarse, squeaky squeeze toys, and items with other textures. Water play can be a lot of fun, as can the sandbox. Toys that an infant can activate with a switch or handle, such as a barking dog, help to teach cause and effect. Use your imagination, and talk to other parents.

Lastly, remember that even the most mundane, workaday outing can be a thrilling and educational experience for your infant or toddler. A visit to the mall or the grocery store becomes an exciting feast for the senses, providing an opportunity to see, feel, and hear the new and unfamiliar. If your little explorer has difficulty getting out into the world, bring the world to her!

The Value of Early Intervention

Twenty-five years ago, young children with a range of developmental problems, including spina bifida, usually faced an isolated, homebound existence or were placed in often inadequate custodial care facilities. In the 1960s, many early childhood demonstration projects were established to address the needs of special infants and toddlers. With the enactment of several public laws, early-intervention projects have become firmly established in all states. Federal incentives are available to encourage states to develop family-centered, community-based services for infants and toddlers. Similar trends have occurred in Canada, Europe, and elsewhere. I will address the issues in greater depth in Chapter 11, in which we will focus on the needs of the child with spina bifida in the educational system.

The enormous volume of research regarding early intervention has shown that such services do indeed enhance the development of infants and toddlers at risk of developmental problems. Young children who have had the benefit of early intervention are more competent and show significant improvements in their behavior. Moreover, there is evidence that families of these children benefit too in terms of their confidence and adaptation to having a young child with special needs. The essential ingredients of such early-intervention programs are (1) a strong commitment to family goals and family support, (2) the identification of the parent as the key person who can influence the child's development, and (3) the provision of a comprehensive and flexible array of services, including home visits, supportive counseling to the parents, and center-based therapy.

As shown in Figure 6.2, early intervention transcends the boundaries of treatment, education, and play. It is stimulating, enjoyable, and rewarding for parent and child. To be successful, it must be integrated into the daily routines of family life. As such, early intervention has to be flexible and take account of family responsibilities and parental goals and perceptions. Parents are necessarily partners in the process. There was one recent occasion where I and other professionals held the opinion that a particular toddler needed intensive, center-based early intervention, but the parent steadfastly refused and did not follow through with treatment plans. This led to frustration and a potential breakdown in the parent-professional

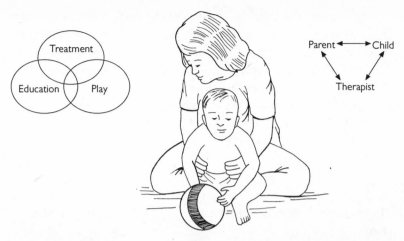

Figure 6.2. Early intervention transcends the boundaries of treatment, education, and play. It is a flexible and dynamic process involving the child, parent, and therapist.

partnership. Under these circumstances, we professionals must remember that early intervention is not a prescribed medical treatment, and it cannot be done in a vacuum. If we encounter resistance, we need to explore the reasons for the divergent perspectives and the real needs of the family. Only by such mutual participation and joint problem solving can we arrive at a satisfactory service plan. In this case, the mother and the local therapist had had some interpersonal problem so that ongoing therapy with this person was clearly not a viable prospect. Once we determined the obstacle, we were able to find alternative therapy arrangements which were acceptable to the mother and from which the toddler clearly benefited.

Frequently, I hear parents voice their dissatisfaction with the quality of the early-intervention services they are receiving, for which there may be many reasons. One common reason for frustration on the part of the parents is lack of progress. Expectations for rapid progress may be high; development is a slow process that does not occur evenly but often imperceptibly or with long periods of stagnation. This leads to disappointment and frustration with the therapist, sometimes unfairly. Also, it is important for the therapy to be proactive and goal directed. Therapy too often proceeds with regular visits but unclear goals or insufficient flexibility. Parents and therapists should work together and be willing to make short-term objectives, adjusting therapy and schedules as necessary to accomplish these objectives.

Furthermore, the financial burden to the family of paying for early-intervention services can be extremely high. Although some costs may be covered by insurance and programs for children with chronic illnesses, most families incur large out-of-pocket expenses (Rosenfeld 1994). As the organization of health care changes dramatically in the United States, middle-class families, especially those with special needs, are being squeezed more tightly, which forces them to make very difficult choices about early-intervention services.

HABILITATION ISSUES

The key issues addressed in this section are mobility, toileting, and nutrition.

Mobility

The Team Approach

Decisions regarding bracing, walking, physical therapy, and orthopedic surgery can be very complex. No two children are exactly alike, and although the basic principles may be reasonably clear, special considerations sometimes influence timing and therapeutic choices. Rational decision making in this vital area of habilitation depends on the expertise of several professionals. Different centers vary in the way these teams are constituted and the manner in which they divide responsibilities. Typically, the team includes an orthopedic surgeon, a physical therapist, and a bioengineering/orthotics specialist. In some centers, a physician who specializes in physical medicine and rehabilitation is a key player.

The Benefits of Early Walking

Although there has long been controversy over whether it is helpful to vigorously assist toddlers with thoracic spina bifida to walk, most of the evidence seems to indicate that there are real benefits. Mazur et al. (1989) found that children with thoracic or high-lumbar spina bifida who were ambulatory—using a combination of extensive bracing, intensive physical therapy, and surgery when needed—had fewer fractures and pressure sores and improvements in bowel and bladder function. Moreover, they were more independent for transfers (from bed to chair, etc.) and some other activities of daily living (Figure 6.3). Most centers, therefore, do what needs to be done to get toddlers upright and walking, albeit with the realization that a large proportion of those children with high lesions will give up walking in favor of their wheelchairs in the years to come.

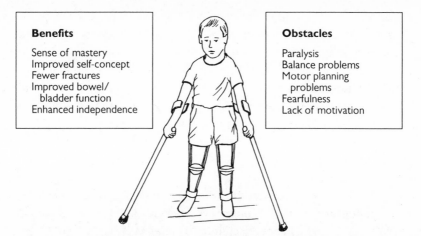

Benefits		Obstacles

Sense of mastery
Improved self-concept
Fewer fractures
Improved bowel/
    bladder function
Enhanced independence
		Paralysis
		Balance problems
		Motor planning
		    problems
		Fearfulness
		Lack of motivation

Figure 6.3. Learning to walk, and some of the benefits of and commonly encountered obstacles to early walking

Obstacles to Walking

Although certainly important, paralysis of the leg muscles is not the only obstacle to walking that needs to be considered. For some young children, balance is significantly impaired because of vestibular or cerebellar deficits. Toddlers with severe balance problems have a history of delayed development of head control, and they show difficulty making postural adjustments when seated, falling easily. Other children have motor planning problems (dyspraxia), initiating a sequence of movements necessary for walking with difficulty. Such toddlers may have speech problems or have trouble self-feeding or imitating such simple gestures as clapping hands. A few children with spina bifida have very significant arm and trunk weakness as a result of associated neurologic dysfunction. For these children, the strength and coordination may be lacking to manage a walker, crutches, or even the trunk movements necessary to initiate walking. Indeed, some of them may not ultimately develop sufficient arm function to move themselves independently in a manual wheelchair.

Another essential prerequisite for walking is the motivation to walk. For almost all toddlers with spina bifida, this comes naturally (although to varying degrees). Many children who appear "lazy" actually have balance problems and a fear of falling. Some young children, however, are very delayed in their development and do not show such motivation. I provide medical care for a girl who is eight years old, severely retarded, and totally dependent for mobility and other needs. She relies on her mother and father for all her feeding, dressing, and bathing needs. Undoubtedly, she has some of the problems mentioned above, but her teacher, physical therapist, and I believe that she has the ability to do more than she currently does for herself. Although it may be too late to bring about any meaningful change for this girl, the key to progress in this kind of situation is finding the thing that motivates behavior. It may be food, it may be a toy, or it may be a Barney video, but something must be found that is worth working for. Progress toward becoming a motivated child comes in small steps and has to begin when the child is very young!

Bracing Needs

Braces, also known as orthoses, are used for three purposes: to assist in standing and walking; to prevent contractures and deformities; and to protect limbs and skin from fractures and injury. Many children with low-level spina bifida have the muscle strength to walk quite well without braces, but the braces are required to keep their feet and ankles in proper alignment while walking in order to prevent further damage and deformity as they grow.

To be useful in walking, the braces have to fulfill certain criteria. They must permit a child to move with relative efficiency and low energy expenditure and at a reasonable speed. Also, they should allow a child to make transfers independently, ultimately permitting him or her to doff and don independently—that is, to put the braces on and take them off by oneself. The design and fit of the braces is very important, as is the systematic training that a child must receive to use the bracing effectively. The orthotist usually takes careful measurements and casts to obtain accurate dimensions of the legs. Once the braces have been made, they are checked and adjusted if necessary before the child takes them home. The physical therapist is instrumental in training a child in the functional skills necessary for assisted ambulation, including don and doff, rolling over, getting to stand, and getting in and out of the wheelchair. Parents and therapists may be additionally helpful in developing the requisite skills for successful use of braces.

The absence of sensation poses special risks for the child with spina bifida who uses braces. If the pressure from the braces is not distributed evenly, the potential exists for rubbing, breakdown, and ulceration of skin. This is especially likely to occur with new braces, because minor irregularities or pressure points may not be appreciated when the braces are first fitted. The braces should be worn for short periods of time initially (one to two hours) so that a child can gradually develop tolerance as the skin toughens and adjusts to the fit. During these early weeks, it is especially

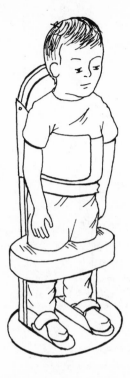

Figure 6.4. The standing frame: an inexpensive device that enables a toddler to stand with an erect posture

important that the parents inspect the skin for areas of reddening or irritation. If the redness persists for twenty to thirty minutes after the braces have been removed or if blistering or skin breakdown occurs, the braces should not be worn until they have been checked by the physical therapist, orthotics specialist, or orthopedic surgeon. The problems of skin care will be discussed in greater depth in Chapter 8.

As in other areas of treatment, braces have undergone significant improvement in recent years, resulting in newer, more efficient designs, lighter materials, and an improved ability to individualize orthotic designs to match the needs of specific children. There are many different designs and styles of bracing, and different clinics have their own preferences. Some clinics even offer designer colors. The orthoses that I describe here are among the more commonly prescribed braces that your toddler may encounter. We begin with the kinds of braces that are typically used in toddlers aged twelve to fifteen months to help them to be upright.

The Standing Frame. The standing brace is a simple device that supports the trunk and legs, enabling a toddler to stand with an erect posture while getting used to the feeling of being upright (Figure 6.4). It is inexpensive and easy to fit. Although it does not have hinges to permit sitting and does

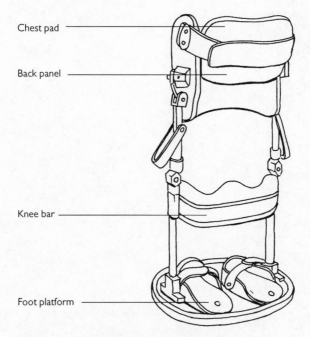

Chest pad

Back panel

Knee bar

Foot platform

Figure 6.5. The parapodium: a brace with a wide base that allows forward movement, usually with a walker or crutches. It is hinged to permit sitting.

not allow a child to move forward, it does afford a child a good opportunity to work on fine-motor and hand manipulation skills.

The Parapodium. The parapodium features a wide base that allows the young child to stand erect without hand support (Figure 6.5). It enables forward movement through a side-to-side movement of the upper body or, more common, with the aid of a walker or crutches (the so-called swing-to gait, in which the child swings the legs together up to the walker and then extends the walker forward for the next step). The parapodium has hinges at the hips and knees; thus the child can sit while in the orthosis. The main disadvantage of the parapodium is that it requires considerable energy expenditure, and children tend to tire easily. Movement is slow and requires a level floor. For toddlers with high lesions who are just beginning to ambulate and for those with balance problems, however, the parapodium is a suitable choice, and most take to it with excitement.

The Swivel Walker. The swivel walker is a rigid brace also used primarily for children with thoracic-level spina bifida who have little or no hip flex-

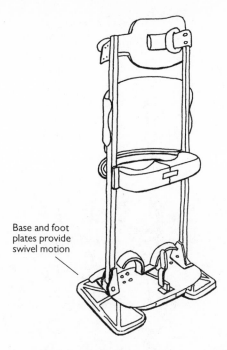

Base and foot
plates provide
swivel motion

Figure 6.6. The swivel walker (ORLAU brace), which enables forward movement with a swivel action

ion (Figure 6.6). It was designed at the Orthotic Research and Locomotion Assessment Unit in Shropshire, England; hence it is also called the ORLAU brace. It encourages early standing and permits walking without crutches or a walker. The young child uses the brace by shifting body weight from side to side, allowing the foot plates to rise alternately and rotate forward. Although the swivel walker is also inefficient and does not allow much speed, it is robust. Moreover, it can also be used in combination with crutches or a walker with a swing-to gait. The principal disadvantage of the swivel walker is that there are no joints at the hips or knees, which makes sitting impossible. Also, it is heavier and more expensive than the parapodium.

The Reciprocating Gait Orthosis (RGO). The RGO is a sophisticated brace that is more commonly used in children with high-level spina bifida who are beyond the toddler years (Figure 6.7). Frequently, it is preceded by the use of the hip-knee-ankle-foot orthosis described below, parapodium, or swivel walker. It has a cable coupling system connecting the two leg supports. When the child leans forward and to the side, the cable system causes the opposite leg to swing forward, thereby enabling reciprocal walking, in which one leg is planted while the other swings. Walking with the RGO is slow but requires relatively little energy. The RGO articulates

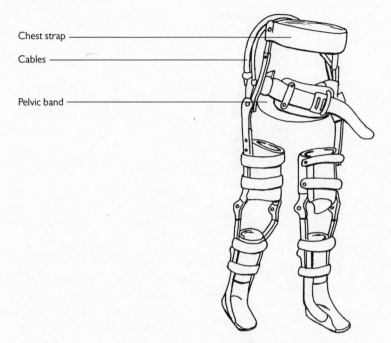

Chest strap

Cables

Pelvic band

Figure 6.7. The reciprocating gait orthosis (RGO). The RGO has a cable system that allows children with good balance to walk with a reciprocal gait—that is, legs move alternately, not together.

at the hips and knees to allow sitting. A child must have good balance and little fear of falling to use the RGO.

Hip-Knee-Ankle-Foot Orthosis (HKAFO). The HKAFO is a metal brace consisting of stainless steel or aluminum long leg braces, with cuffs around the thighs and calves, and a pelvic band (Figure 6.8). For children with poor trunk control, an additional corset can be added for the trunk (THKAFO). The orthosis is used with crutches or a walker, and the gait may be either swing-to or swing-through (the child swings both legs past the crutches). The long leg braces are easily adjustable, with joints that can be unlocked for sitting or other purposes.

Knee-Ankle-Foot Orthosis (KAFO). For children who have sufficient hip flexors and do not require the pelvic band, KAFOs are frequently used (Figure 6.9). These long leg braces are usually made of polypropylene, which has many advantages. They are lighter and less obtrusive and can be worn inside regular shoes. In addition to their use for walking, these braces can also serve an important stretching function.

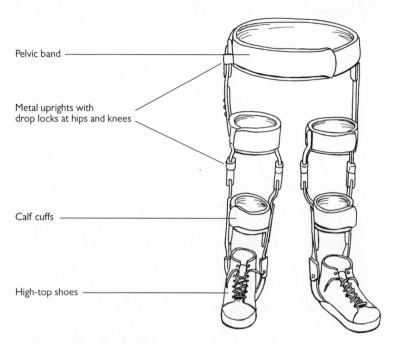

Pelvic band

Metal uprights with
drop locks at hips and knees

Calf cuffs

High-top shoes

Figure 6.8. Long leg braces (HKAFO), which are easily adjustable for use with a walker or crutches

Short Leg Braces/Ankle-Foot Orthosis (AFO). AFOs are used for children who have adequate muscle control of the hip and the knee joint but not at the ankle (Figure 6.10). They can be made of metal with a leather calf cuff and a direct attachment to an orthopedic shoe but these days are more commonly made of polypropylene. For older, heavier children, carbon fibers are corrugated into the brace to add strength. The polypropylene AFO is molded to the lower leg and can be inserted into the back of a regular shoe. The brace provides support around the ankle joint and can be designed to counteract existing deformity and to maintain normal alignment of the ankle and foot. Polypropylene AFOs are lighter than the metal ones and can maintain good alignment. There tends to be more perspiration, however, so it is important to watch for skin problems. These days, AFOs and other polypropylene orthoses are available in fashionable designer colors!

Some children may experience a lot of rotation at the hip, with feet in an abnormal position and particularly out-toeing as a result of this external rotation. AFOs do not correct for these rotational problems; thus pelvic bands with twister cables are sometimes necessary.

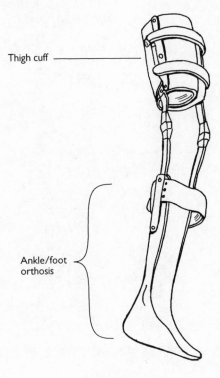

Thigh cuff

Ankle/foot
orthosis

Figure 6.9. Long leg braces
(KAFO), commonly used by
children with hip flexion but
insufficient knee extension

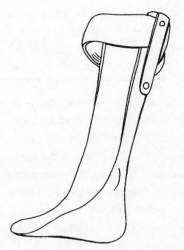

Figure 6.10. Short leg brace/ankle-
foot orthosis (AFO): lightweight
polypropylene braces provide support
around the ankles.

LORENZ NIGHT SPLINT

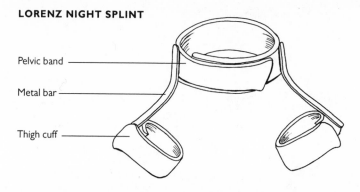

Pelvic band

Metal bar

Thigh cuff

DENIS-BROWNE SPLINT

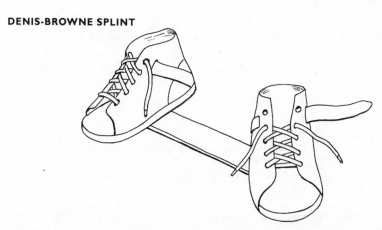

Figure 6.11. The abduction splint (Lorenz night splint) helps to prevent hip dislocation. The Denis-Browne splint can be used in the treatment of clubfoot deformities, as well as in the treatment of hip dysplasia.

Splints. The Pope night splint is a simple splint that is worn at night by infants and toddlers with tight heel cords in order to prevent contractures. They are usually set to maintain the ankles at ninety degrees. Casting can be used for the same effect but has the disadvantage of immobilizing the foot during the day. These night splints are usually worn for a few months, in conjunction with physical therapy, to maintain range of motion.

The abduction splint is designed to prevent hip dislocation (Figure 6.11). By maintaining the legs in an abducted position, the head of the femur is kept in contact with the socket of the hip joint. The device is worn at night and during naps to obtain maximum effect.

The Denis-Browne splint consists of a bar with two shoes attached. It is used in young children with high lesions to minimize the development of

Lofstrand crutches

Walker

Rollator

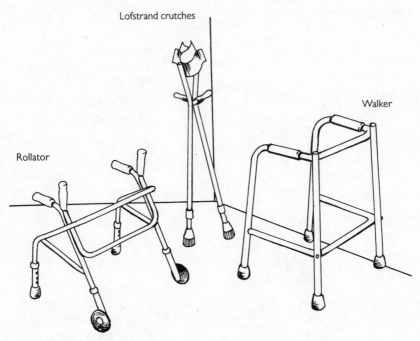

Figure 6.12. Crutches and walkers: these robust walking aids need to be monitored for wear and tear.

hip external rotation/abduction contractures. It may also be used in the treatment of clubfeet, to counteract the abnormal positioning of the feet. The length of the bar can be adjusted, and the size, position, and shape of the shoe can be varied to suit the needs of the infant.

Crutches and Walkers. Many toddlers who walk with braces are able to balance well with crutches. These are usually the Lofstrand type, which attach to the forearm, rather than the longer crutches which fit in the armpit (Figure 6.12). Lofstrand crutches are robust and long-lasting but need to be checked for wear. The rubber tips must be in good condition to prevent slipping and dangerous falls. For many young children, however, balance problems and insecurity make the use of a rollator walker preferable in the early stages of walking. These provide greater support than crutches but are not as easily maneuverable. Walkers must be monitored for signs of wear and tear, and their length may need adjustment as the child grows. Generally, the handles of the walker should be around the level of the hips, so the elbows are flexed to about thirty degrees when the child is holding them.

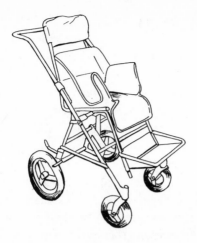

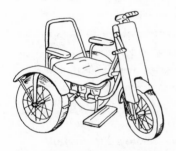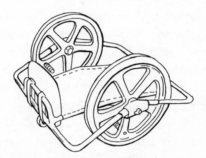

Figure 6.13. Wheeled mobility devices such as scooter boards and Star cars can help toddlers develop strength and coordination, while getting around independently.

Other Mobility Aids. Some toddlers learn to be independently mobile in a small wheelchair. However, the emphasis in this age group is on attaining upright mobility, and I have therefore saved my discussion of wheelchairs until Chapter 7. There are a number of wheeled mobility devices that can be particularly helpful in this age group (Figure 6.13). For instance, the scooter board allows a toddler to propel herself safely and effectively with her hands alone while lying low to the ground in a prone position. Similarly, the Star car is ideally suited to the active child with spina bifida who lacks the muscles for upright mobility, also providing valuable early experience and training in how to use a wheelchair. Such mobility aids may contribute to a child's strength, coordination, motor planning, and body awareness, enabling her to explore her environment independently.

Physical and Sensorimotor Therapy

As I noted, early intervention is clearly beneficial for infants and toddlers with spina bifida. Different therapists have different techniques and philosophies, and the needs of individual children are so variable; thus it is impossible to describe an exact recipe for success. In my view, the key ingredient in a successful program of physical and sensorimotor therapy is a clear focus on function rather than any adherence to a rigid dogma. The interdependence of different aspects of early child development should be stressed. For example, fine-motor skills may be enhanced by achieving the gross-motor milestone of a stable sit. Also important to remember is that children frequently do not follow the typical sequences of development; thus the absence of crawling should not preclude therapeutic efforts directed toward balance, posture, and standing. In our clinic, the physical therapist and occupational therapist work together closely, enhancing functional skills through their integrated efforts spanning the areas of gross-motor, fine-motor, adaptive, and cognitive development.

The therapists should conduct ongoing assessments of the infant. Specific functional impairments, such as poor sitting balance, should be identified in order for these areas to be addressed through therapy. As therapy progresses, the infant achieves the short-term functional goal, and in so doing, a new functional impairment emerges as the next focus for ongoing therapy. In this way, ever-advancing, short-term goals are set, and the infant or toddler makes stepwise progress toward improved motor function and mobility. The book by Williamson (1987) is particularly useful in illustrating the kinds of sensorimotor interventions that are most helpful. Figure 6.14 illustrates a few important short-term therapy goals, some of the components used to achieve them, and the long-term implications for improving the child's functional skills.

This approach is best illustrated by considering an infant with spina bifida at around six months of age. Let's say the infant has good head control in a supported sit but is unable to maintain sitting balance. She sits with her legs straight out in front, and her trunk falls forward almost onto her legs or out to the side when she is not supported. The key neurologic impairment here is poor trunk control and weak abdominal muscles. The therapist can help to strengthen these muscles by bottom lifting (when the infant lies on her back and the therapist helps her to bring hands and feet together, lifting the bottom up off the mat) and also by encouraging head and neck flexion when she is prone (on her belly) on her extended arms. Postural control in the sitting position can be enhanced by holding her in supported sit, keeping her pelvis forward, and displacing her weight

Therapy is directed to improving long-term functional skills

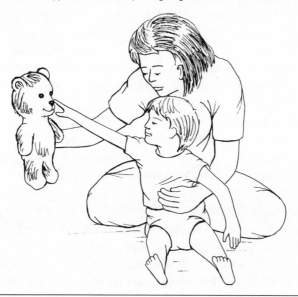

Short-term therapy goals	Components of therapy to achieve goals	Long-term functional skills
Tool use (shovel, spoon, crayon, mallet)	Hand strength Force gradation Tactile input Perception Proper orientation of tool Eye-hand coordination	Handwriting Toothbrushing Catheterization Use of scissors
Transfer on/off a small bench	Upper body/trunk strengthening Spatial perception/ body awareness Balance Propulsion of body Motor planning and organization	Transfers from wheelchair, floor, bed, toilet Prerequisite for ambulation
Visual scanning of environment	Depth perception Figure-ground discrimination Object discrimination Visual memory and attention	Visual orientation for mobility School performance Safety
Simple dressing (removing shoes, socks, shirt)	Body part orientation Body scheme Grasp patterns Bilateral coordination Balance	Working toward independent dressing

Figure 6.14. Selected short-term therapy goals may help a child develop long-term functional skills.

gently backward. It may be helpful to place toys in reach on a table at about the level of the infant's shoulders to motivate the child to maintain a straight trunk. As sitting balance improves, the therapist may wish to focus its enhancement with rotation, encouraging her to reach sideways for toys. The next goal may be the development of sequenced movements, working on the goal of getting from the prone position to sitting and back to prone again.

Rolling from supine to prone (back to front) and then from prone to supine are important early mobility skills that are usually present by around five or six months of age. Rolling is usually a problem for an infant with high-level spina bifida. It may be difficult for him to shift weight, or the positioning of his legs may act as a barrier to the rolling movement. The therapist can work on these skills by playing in the side-lying position and guiding the infant in compensatory movements of the head, arms, and upper trunk that can be used to initiate such rolling movements.

Next, we can consider the older infant, say around nine months of age, who is showing a readiness to crawl on his belly. Most infants with spina bifida are able to bear weight on their elbows and propel themselves forward by reciprocally pulling themselves along with their arms. Those with thoracic spina bifida will usually commando crawl with their legs out behind them, whereas those with active hip flexion may develop a quadriped crawl on their arms and knees. The goal of therapy during the initial development of these mobility skills is to strengthen the arms and help the infant develop reciprocal arm crawling patterns. This goal may be facilitated with the assistance of gravity, encouraging the infant to crawl downhill while on an inclined surface, such as a large wedge. For the infant with active hip flexion, progression from commando crawling to quadriped crawling can be facilitated by helping the child into a quadriped position and initiating gentle rocking movements. Some infants will tend to move the legs together as a unit, developing bunny hopping or scooting forward on the buttocks, rather than developing reciprocal leg movements. Because reciprocal movements are important for the development of normal walking patterns, the therapist can encourage this by extending one leg, so that the child is positioned prone on both arms and one leg. In addition, it can be helpful to get the infant to move from the quadriped position to side sitting and back to the quadriped position.

Some months later, we can consider the challenges for the toddler with spina bifida who is crawling, trying to pull up to the kneeling position, and showing a readiness to stand. Here, the goal of the therapist may be to help her to pull up successfully to the kneeling position. Again, arm and

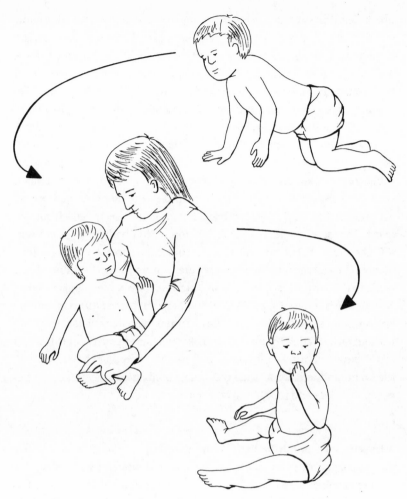

Figure 6.15. Therapy with a nine-month-old child may involve the development of reciprocal leg patterns as the child moves from the quadriped position to side sitting and back to the quadriped position.

trunk strengthening and enhancing trunk control and balance reactions can be very important. In addition, the timely use of braces, crutches, or other aids as previously discussed can help such a child stand and become ready to begin learning to walk.

The Future: Functional Electrical Stimulation

There has long been interest in the development of a system of electrical stimulation of muscles to enhance strength and allow walking. Functional electrical stimulation is particularly relevant in the case of traumatic spinal cord injury, where the muscles are normal and the neuromuscular system is intact until the moment of injury. For spina bifida, there may be very little useful muscle because, in effect, there has never been an intact neuromuscular system, so those affected muscles did not ever develop normally. But the muscles are present and may have the potential to grow and develop to some extent if they are systematically stimulated by electronic means from an early age. Although they may never develop the strength to power a limb, such electrically stimulated muscles could conceivably contribute to mobility. If such a system were combined with orthoses, however, these could maintain the body in equilibrium. An integrated, closed-loop feedback system could electrically stimulate selected muscles (perhaps in combination with a hydraulic system outside the body that is housed in the orthotic) to control walking movements. The system may include pressure sensors in the heel and toe to regulate the movements, and a computerized control mechanism to deal with changes in terrain, balance, and other conditions. Although a long way off, such a system may have the potential to enable efficient mobility without fatigue and excessive arm use. Research into systems of this sort is continuing and may eventually lead to new techniques of habilitation in the infant and toddler. As such technologies advance, the boundaries between orthotics and robotics may dissolve.

Toileting

A Developmental Approach to Toilet Training

The process of toilet training involves the following steps: First, the toddler develops a predictable pattern of behavior and timing in emptying bladder and bowel. Next, the parent recognizes these patterns and responds in a positive and helping way (by changing a diaper, taking her to the potty, and so on). The child then develops more awareness of these processes, in part dependent on the sensory feedback associated with bladder and bowel contractions during elimination. In time, she learns to exert control over these processes of elimination by "holding on," until willfully letting go in the toilet, to the delight of her parents. The process is essentially one of learning and mastery. Through toilet training, the toddler learns the social value of controlling her impulses and emerges with a heightened sense of autonomy and accomplishment. Although the outcome is usually a very positive one in the development of the child, the process is often difficult and frustrating. Parents of children with spina bifida should not get the idea that it is always clear sailing for other kids!

Punitive approaches on the part of the parent are especially likely to derail successful toilet training by conveying a sense of failure and shame to the confused toddler.

For the toddler with spina bifida, issues of toilet training are often overlooked. Perhaps the child's pediatrician might have said, "Oh, he has no sensation of bladder and bowel so there's no point in trying to toilet train him. Just wait until he's older and then we can get him on a program and manage his bladder and bowel for him." Certainly, sensations of bladder and bowel fullness or contractions are impaired or absent, but some sensation may be present and may raise the toddler's awareness of elimination. Moreover, the other important prerequisites for toilet training are indeed present for the child with spina bifida. In other words, he usually develops a pattern or schedule that his parents can recognize and respond to appropriately. I believe that toilet training has benefits for the child with spina bifida. While sitting on the toilet, gravity assists in bowel and bladder emptying. Moreover, it is a normal experience that can be fun for a toddler.

For example, a typical, nearly two-year-old girl with spina bifida had bowel movements once or twice a day, usually after breakfast or after the evening meal (this is a result of the gastrocolic reflex, whereby a full stomach triggers contractions of the colon and stimulates emptying of the rectum). Her parents saw the regularity of this pattern and learned to recognize the cessation of activity and slight reddening of her cheeks as she strained a little. They commented on this simply and in a positive way to their daughter, and then promptly changed her diaper. She seemed interested and aware of this routine, and when they gave her a potty for her birthday, she enjoyed sitting on it. I suggested that they put her on the potty if they thought she was about to have a bowel movement. They began by sitting her on the potty for a few minutes after each meal. Indeed, there were many occasions when her parents timed it just right and she deposited stool in the right place! There were even a few occasions when she took the initiative to go to her chair and take off her diaper. In any event, she took responsibility for helping to change her diaper and clean herself. More important, the positive responses of her parents communicated their pride in her accomplishment. Now, at age four, she is learning how to bear down or strain actively (the Valsalva maneuver). Even though she will not develop normal bowel control, I think the chances are excellent that she will achieve continence.

As this vignette illustrates, toilet training is an important opportunity for a toddler to learn the social value of continence and to master new

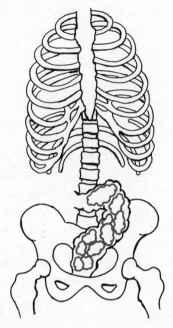

**Complications
of constipation**

Anal fissures
Skin breakdown
Poor appetite
Incontinence
Intestinal obstruction
Urinary tract infection

Figure 6.16. Constipation in young children as shown by the distended colon on an X-ray, and the complications of constipation

skills autonomously. For the toddler with spina bifida, there may have to be modifications in the methods or the expectations because of his or her neurologic impairments. Handled with sensitivity, the experience can still be a valuable one, laying a solid foundation for subsequent development of continence.

Avoiding Constipation

Infants and toddlers with spina bifida are very prone to constipation. It is important to remember that constipation really refers to the consistency of the stool rather than to the number of times a child passes stool. The hallmark of constipation is hard stool. The infant who passes hard balls of stool three times a day is still constipated. Typically, the constipated child has a lot of stool in the colon, some of which may be hard, and some soft. The stool may often be felt, especially in the lower abdomen on the left side. If X-rays are taken for some reason—for example, to examine the hips—we frequently see large amounts of stool extending from the rectum along most of the length of the colon (Figure 6.16).

The prevention of constipation is of great importance in the early years because it can be difficult or impossible to recondition a bowel that

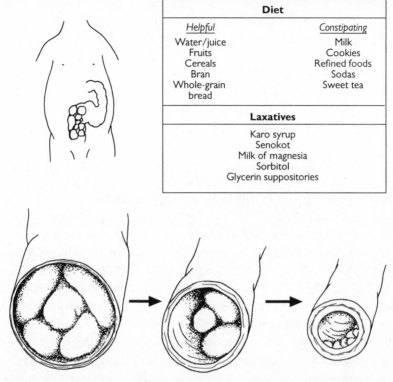

Diet	
Helpful	*Constipating*
Water/juice	Milk
Fruits	Cookies
Cereals	Refined foods
Bran	Sodas
Whole-grain bread	Sweet tea

Laxatives
Karo syrup
Senokot
Milk of magnesia
Sorbitol
Glycerin suppositories

Figure 6.17. Preventing constipation: dietary measures may be sufficient to maintain soft and regular stools, but laxative therapy may be required to help clear a large, distended colon.

has been stretched for years by the accumulation of hard stool. In its most severe form, constipation can lead to blockage of the bowel from fecal impaction. More commonly constipation causes a number of medical problems, including fissuring and abscess formation around the anus, recurrent urinary tract infections, and poor appetite. Moreover, chronic constipation can make the attainment of fecal continence much more difficult. Therefore, it is essential to pay close attention to the bowel within the first few months—and to continue to do so throughout early childhood.

It is almost always possible to prevent and manage constipation in infancy by dietary means. Most parents usually discover what works best and are able to keep the baby's stools soft and consistent. Figure 6.17 illustrates some suggestions for preventing constipation in infants and toddlers. The most important thing is to make sure that the child receives enough fluids. Offer water or unsweetened fruit juice every two hours (the daily requirement of fluid is around one to two quarts). The addition of Karo syrup to her formula (one to two teaspoons per four-ounce bottle) is useful. When she is old enough to eat baby foods, experiment with such "p" fruits as pears, plums, prunes, and peaches. For the toddler, try different cereals, especially those with high bran content, and breads with whole grains. At the same time, it is often helpful to cut back on certain foods in the diet that may be increasing the constipation, such as milk, refined breads and cereals, cookies, and candy.

Stool softeners and stimulant laxatives may have a role to play for some toddlers with constipation that persists despite dietary measures. When used appropriately, these can be very effective and safe. One or two teaspoons of mineral oil (which is available in palatable preparations) may be added after supper. Milk of magnesia tends to act as a stimulant of the bowel and may be helpful in small doses of one-half to one teaspoon twice a day. Available in liquid or granules, Senokot is a natural stimulant that may also be useful for toddlers with constipation. It may be necessary to begin occasional use of glycerin suppositories in toddlers with a lot of hard stool impacted in the rectum. The use of suppositories and enemas is typically delayed until around school entry, however, when such measures become important components of a bowel program to establish and maintain continence. I shall therefore discuss the topic of bowel programs in Chapter 8.

Nutrition and Prevention of Obesity

The plotting of height and weight on the growth curves is one of the most important things for me to do in the spina bifida clinic. Excessive weight gain in infancy or during the toddler years usually leads to obesity in later life, and as we shall see, the prevention of obesity is one of the keys to better health among adolescents and adults with spina bifida (Figure 6.18). Our eating habits are established early in life to a large extent. Convincing scientific evidence also indicates that early obesity affects the body's subsequent metabolism and the way in which fat cells are distributed. There is no getting away from it: the solution to this multifaceted problem lies in the first years of life.

There are many reasons why I have to watch those growth curves carefully and discuss my concerns with parents. Children with spina bifida usually have lower calorie requirements because of muscle weakness and inactivity. They also have a tendency to be short for their age; thus extra fat is more apparent. Sometimes, parents or grandparents love their chil-

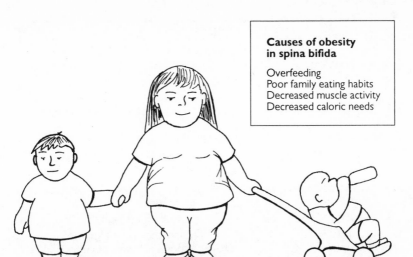

**Causes of obesity
in spina bifida**

Overfeeding
Poor family eating habits
Decreased muscle activity
Decreased caloric needs

Figure 6.18. The causes and consequences of obesity in early life. The child with spina bifida has decreased caloric needs, and poor family eating habits may make obesity a family affair.

dren so much that they can't say no, and the overwhelming love they feel somehow gets attached to the delicious (high-calorie) food they offer. When an infant gains more than five ounces per week, or a kilogram (two pounds) in two months, it's usually time to go on a diet!

There are no magic solutions or shortcuts to good nutrition and the prevention of obesity. The bottom line is that the child needs to eat sufficient good, nutritious food, while eating less high-calorie food of lower nutritional value. The value of aerobic exercise will be addressed in Chapter 9.

When it comes to working out a meal plan for your toddler, use the four basic food groups—that is, meat; milk; vegetables and fruits; and breads, cereals, and starches. The meat group includes meat, fish, poultry, eggs, beans, and nuts (high-protein foods). The milk group includes milk and other dairy products such as cheese and yogurt. Figure 6.19 shows the daily servings and amounts of foods that would constitute a balanced diet for a child between the ages of one and five years. There are many valuable resources for nutritional advice, including your pediatrician's office or local health department. For most families, however, a few common-sense tips shown in the figure may be very helpful in preventing obesity in the child with spina bifida (and promoting healthy nutrition for the whole family).

Servings	Food group	Examples of 1 serving
4	Milk/cheese	½ cup (4 ounces) milk or yogurt 1 ounce cheese
2	Meat	1 ounce beef, chicken, or fish ¼ cup cottage cheese or dried beans 1 egg 1 tablespoon peanut butter
4	Fruits/vegetables	½ cup of citrus, berries, or cantaloupe 3 tablespoons of other fruits or vegetables
4	Breads/cereals/starch	⅓ cup cooked cereal ½ cup dry cereal ⅓ cup spaghetti, rice, or potato
3	Fats	1 teaspoon or pat of margarine 1 tablespoon oil/mayonnaise

Breakfast: Milk, Bread, Fat   Snack: Fruit
Lunch: Milk, Vegetable, Meat, Bread, Fat   Snack: Fruit
Dinner: Milk, Vegetable, Meat, Bread, Fat   Snack: Fruit

Figure 6.19. Daily meal plan for a two- or three-year-old child with spina bifida

Medical Issues

The Unstable Hip

Hip flexors and adductors are controlled primarily by L1- and L2-level nerves, whereas hip extensors and abductors are controlled primarily by nerves at levels L5 to S1. This accounts for the high prevalence of hip instability in the young child with spina bifida, as the muscles acting around the hip joint are unbalanced. Indeed, 25 to 50 percent of newborns with high-lumbar or midlumbar lesions have subluxed or dislocated hips, and at least another 25 percent become unstable during the next few years.

There is a progression of abnormality that is illustrated in Figure 6.20. In the normal hip joint, the femoral head is located within a well-formed socket (acetabulum). The changes that are initially evident with muscle imbalance are known as hip dysplasia, in which the acetabulum does not form its normal deep cup, and the femoral head is at risk of dislocation. Subluxation refers to the partial uncovering of the femoral head by a shallow dysplastic acetabulum. A subluxated hip can be manually reduced (that is, positioned so that the femoral head returns to its proper position abutting the acetabulum) by holding the hip in flexion and abduction. The last stage in the progression of hip instability is the dislocated hip, in which the

Normal

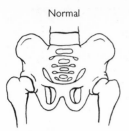

Subluxed

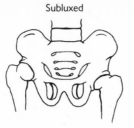

Dislocated

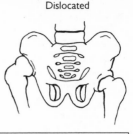

Figure 6.20. Hip instability, showing progression from normal to subluxed to dislocated right hip, and typical associated clinical findings

Typical clinical findings

Decreased hip abduction
Asymmetry
Leg length discrepancy
Extra skin folds
Ortolani test—relocates
Barlow test—dislocatable

femoral head is no longer abutting the acetabulum, lying instead above and behind the socket. The typical signs of dislocation on physical examination are also shown in Figure 6.20. There is usually decreased abduction. There may also be asymmetry in the contour of the hip, as well as extra skin folds in the perineal region because of apparent shortening of the limb. In addition, the Ortolani test (the manual reduction of a dislocated hip) and the Barlow test (the dislocation of a dislocatable hip) may be positive. The most useful investigations are plain X-rays of the pelvis.

The main concern about the dislocated hip is not the effects on walking. In fact, the structural integrity of the hip joint is not required for an adequate swing gait (Menelaus 1980). The real danger lies in asymmetric hips, which causes the pelvis to lie at an angle. The development of pelvic tilt can in turn lead to scoliosis. In addition, it can make seating difficult and predispose the child to pressure sores because pressure is not evenly distributed across the pelvis. For these reasons, it is beneficial to intervene early.

The mainstay of early-intervention efforts is physical therapy to prevent hip contractures. Flexion and adduction contractures of the hips are the most common among children with midlevel spina bifida, whereas higher levels are more often associated with abduction/external rotation contractures. Therapy for these latter children is particularly aimed at stretching the tight ligaments on the outer aspect of the thighs (iliotibial band). The goal is to prevent fixed flexion and adduction deformities at

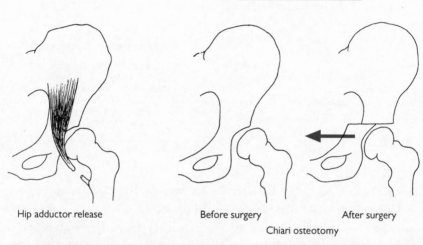

Goals of surgery

Correct deformity
Restore muscle balance
Obtain full extension
Decrease asymmetry
Improve ambulation

Hip adductor release

Before surgery   After surgery

Chiari osteotomy

Figure 6.21. Surgical treatment of hip problems: adductor release and Chiari osteotomy procedures, with likely goals of proceeding with surgery

the hips, which may severely impair later efforts to walk with an upright posture and which can also make catheterization very challenging.

Among the conservative interventions that may be helpful during the first two years are the Pavlik harness, the Lorenz night splint, the Frejka pillow splint, and the hip spica cast. These devices all aim to maintain the hip in the position of manual reduction—in other words, with the hips flexed and abducted. In this way, the joint is encouraged to develop a normal shape, and deforming forces are opposed. The splints are usually worn during sleep and naps, whereas the spica cast cannot be taken off. The problem with these treatments is that they interfere with the development of early mobility skills.

There are a number of surgical treatments for hip problems (Figure 6.21). For the most part, the purpose of surgery is to correct joint contracture and bony deformity, to restore muscle balance around the hip joint, to allow full extension of the hip, and to decrease asymmetry. For children with strong quadriceps function who are likely to learn to walk well an additional goal is to improve walking. As a general rule, most orthopedic surgeons like to do only one operation per hip joint to prevent hip stiffness.

If hip flexion/adductor contractures do occur and interfere with bracing, some form of surgical hip release is usually done. This may involve an adductor release, in which the tendons of the adductors are cut. Alternatively, the nerve to the adductor muscles may be partially excised (obturator neurectomy). If additional stability and symmetry of muscle function is sought, the surgeon may perform some form of tendon transfer. For example, the external oblique abdominal muscle may be moved to insert on the posterior aspect of the greater trochanter. This will counter the forces of the unopposed hip flexors and adductors. Typically, children who have this kind of operation are hospitalized for three to five days and are in casts for four weeks.

Different forms and degrees of severity of the unstable hip in spina bifida require different surgical approaches. Among the more complex operations are those that are designed to improve the alignment of the hip joint itself. The Chiari osteotomy is intended to deepen the hip socket by cutting across the pelvis just above the acetabulum and moving the bone to create a deeper rim for the femoral head. Another option is to cut across the femur and rotate it to realign the femoral head into the acetabulum (varus derotation osteotomy). Both operations require about three or four days in hospital and are followed by casting for four to six weeks. While the children are in casts, they are encouraged to stand, for prolonged immobilization leads to osteoporosis.

Shunt Function and Malfunction

These days, improvements in shunt technology and surgical techniques allow us to be optimistic about shunt function. More than half of all newborn recipients of ventriculo-peritoneal shunts have no significant episodes of shunt malfunction and keep the same shunt until late childhood, at which time the shunt tubing may need lengthening to accommodate increasing growth. About 40 percent of children do require a shunt revision, however, and some of these go on to need subsequent revisions. The peak age at which shunt failure occurs is in the first year of life, although shunt problems can occur at any age, even in an adolescent or adult who is thought to be "not shunt-dependent." Thus the discussion of shunt failure in this chapter has relevance for all ages. Unfortunately, it is impossible to predict which children are going to have shunt problems along the way. It is understandable, given this uncertainty, that many parents feel extremely anxious about their child's shunt. Although excessive vigilance and worry is not going to do anyone any good, it is essential to know about the signs of shunt failure.

As in most aspects of pediatrics, good decision making depends on accurate measurement. Measuring the infant's head circumference and plotting the measurement on a chart remains one of the most valuable clinical tools. As long as the sutures of the skull bones have not fused, the head circumference remains a very reliable indicator of the status of the ventricles. If the shunt is obstructed, the ventricles increase in size, and the head circumference grows faster than it normally would. Figure 5.9 shows how to measure the circumference. It is important to measure the widest occipital-frontal head circumference, if necessary getting an assistant to hold the tape in place if it keeps slipping. Make sure the tape is even and not twisted and that barrettes and other hair decorations are not getting in the way. I always measure at least twice and take the longer of the two measurements. Then plot the measurement accurately on the head circumference chart.

The signs of raised intracranial pressure are usually not very subtle in the infant and toddler. In addition to the rapid increase in head circumference, several other signs may be evident. The anterior fontanel, or "soft spot" (which is usually still open at around twelve months of age), may be unusually full or bulging. The sutures may feel slightly split. The shunt track should be examined closely for evidence of swelling or redness, and the shunt tubing should be carefully felt for any evidence of disconnection. Small veins on the forehead or around the eyes may seem unusually prominent, and the eyes may have a characteristic downward deviation, known as "sunset" appearance. Usually there is no obvious change in mental state or behavior in infants whose sutures have not yet fused, because the skull remains flexible and can therefore accommodate the increasing ventricles without much change in pressure. In severe cases, however, raised intracranial pressure does occur, and the infant may show evidence of breathing problems, cyanosis, or other Chiari-related symptoms. In toddlers and young children, the signs of shunt malfunction may be as subtle as mild drowsiness and impaired coordination. Headache, irritability, and lethargy are the most common signs. Fever, vomiting, and seizures may also occur.

When the symptoms and signs of shunt failure are clearly present or when there is indisputable evidence of ventricular enlargement on the CT scan, the diagnostic issues are clear-cut. Unfortunately, this is not always the case. Symptoms may be subtle and vague, making it hard to know whether the shunt is malfunctioning or the child has a viral infection. Symptoms may be intermittent, as a shunt is temporarily obstructed and then free flowing again. In these puzzling situations, the astute clinician maintains a high index of suspicion of shunt malfunction. This is especially the case if parents who have already had experience of previous shunt malfunction in their child are saying that they think it's the shunt again.

Investigating shunt function requires an experienced neurosurgeon. The most helpful investigation is the unenhanced CT scan, which can be compared with previous films to determine whether ventricular enlargement has occurred.

Many clinicians obtain information about the patency of the shunt by pumping it, that is, depressing the reservoir and letting it refill: a shunt that depresses easily has unobstructed outflow, and the shunt that fills easily has unobstructed inflow from the ventricles. Unfortunately, this simple test has been found to be quite unreliable. The sensitivity (the ability of this test to detect abnormal shunt function) is around only 18–20 percent; thus the clinician cannot be very reassured by a normal shunt pumping test. There is also a small risk that pumping a shunt may actually cause shunt obstruction in a child with a slitlike ventricle. Measuring CSF pressures and flow directly by tapping the shunt can sometimes provide the neurosurgeon with helpful information, as well as affording an opportunity to examine the CSF under the microscope for evidence of infection. Such a test is invasive, however, requires shaving part of the head, and carries a risk of introducing infection. More recently, Moss, Marchbanks, and Burge (1991) described a new technique of assessing intracranial pressure indirectly. This technique is based on the observation that the tympanic membrane in the ear is displaced by loud sound and that this displacement is altered when the intracranial pressure is raised.

Chiari Malformation

The Chiari malformation was discussed in depth in the previous chapter. The symptoms of the infantile form of Chiari malformation may persist into the toddler years, during which it commonly interferes with feeding skills.

At six to twelve months of age, most babies progress from sucking to munching. At the same time, babies develop more control of lip movements, which enables them actively to take food from a spoon and begin to drink from a cup. At twelve to twenty-four months, toddlers develop increasingly complex and coordinated movements of their lips, tongue, and jaw. They learn to drink from a cup without spilling, to handle different textures, and to feed themselves by hand and even with a spoon.

For the toddler with spina bifida and Chiari malformation, this progression of skills may not develop normally. Liquids and food may dribble or pool in the cheeks. There may be a lot of gurgling noises as the child struggles to swallow food, mucus, and saliva. They may always seem to be congested. Many such children have trouble with different textures of food, and their oral hypersensitivity may lead to prominent gagging symptoms, a tendency that may remain even into adulthood. If severe, the Chiari malformation may cause choking, aspiration, recurrent pneumonias, and failure to thrive.

The mechanism of Chiari malformation involves compression of the lower brainstem. Many cranial nerves that are important for feeding and swallowing are found in this area of the brain. They include the nerves that supply the muscles of the mouth and tongue, as well as sensation from the oral areas. In addition to the effects on these important cranial nerves, the Chiari malformation may affect the spinal cord, causing stiff neck, weakness in the arms, and numbness in the hands. Even less common may be compression of the cerebellum, causing unsteadiness (ataxia).

Management of the Chiari malformation depends on the severity of the symptoms. For the infant or toddler with mild oral hypersensitivity and feeding problems, it may be sufficient to work on developing hand-to-mouth and toys-to-mouth skills. Oral stimulation, involving the gentle massaging of gums, lips, tongue, and cheeks, may be helpful in gradually overcoming the hypersensitivity. Adaptations may need to be made to the diet in terms of providing consistent textures that the child can manage easily. In such a child, it is usually possible to progress from pureed foods to thicker foods, such as mashed potato, and then on to lumpier foods, such as rice pudding. Chewy textures may be the most difficult for a child to handle. It is also beneficial to try different temperatures. Pediatric occupational therapists are usually experienced in these aspects of management.

If the symptoms are much more severe, it is usually necessary to do a more extensive workup. This may include a swallowing study or an ear, nose, and throat (ENT) evaluation. Speech therapists and occupational therapists may also contribute to such feeding evaluations and be very helpful in management. Although rare, it may be necessary to provide an alternate way to obtain sufficient calories for adequate nutrition. Temporary feeding tubes that allow drip feeds overnight through a nasogastric tube may be required for short-term nutritional supplements. For children with severe and long-lasting nutritional inadequacy, it is a simple procedure to place a gastrostomy tube that passes directly into the stomach. Such a tube allows parents to give additional high-calorie formula and can be very helpful with growth and development; it may be needed for a few months or a few years, depending on how feeding skills progress. Although a daunting and frightening prospect for all families, they are actually quite easy to manage at home and can be lifesaving in many circumstances of inadequate nutrition.

As always, it is essential to make sure that the shunt is working normally in a child with new symptoms of Chiari malformation. The neurosurgeon will also be involved in the evaluation of the brainstem, using an MRI scan. Operations to decompress the brainstem by cervical laminectomy may relieve Chiari-related symptoms, although this is by no means certain.

Failure to Thrive

On a few occasions, I have encountered very young children with spina bifida who fail to grow and gain weight adequately, although they appear to feed well and have no significant Chiari-related symptoms. Some of these infants may be growing at a normal or near-normal rate, but well below the fifth percentile, whereas others may be falling off their growth curves and genuinely failing to thrive. The causes of failure to thrive are legion, and it is not uncommon for a careful history to reveal evidence of infrequent feeding or unintentional dilution of formula. Another treatable cause is renal tubular acidosis, which may follow prolonged high bladder pressures and neonatal hydronephrosis. It is helpful to check urine pH and serum electrolytes to find evidence of metabolic acidosis. Once the diagnosis is confirmed, the addition of baking soda or Bicitra can normalize the low serum bicarbonate, thereby providing more optimal conditions for growth.

Strabismus

Many children with spina bifida have some difficulty with the coordinated control of eye movements, which for many does not lead to any problems. They can see with normal acuity, but their eye movements are somewhat jerky when they are following objects that are moving in front of them. For some, however, there is squinting (or strabismus), such that the eyes are seen to be crossed (esotropia) or divergent (exotropia). If the squinting is due mainly to one eye, to avoid confusion the brain quite quickly learns to suppress the image coming from the troublesome eye.

This process is called amblyopia, or "lazy eye," and can lead to permanent loss of normal binocular vision. It is important to report concerns about squinting or poor vision to the health care team; an appropriate referral can then be made to an ophthalmologist. Many youngsters with amblyopia can be managed effectively with glasses and the use of patches. If the "good eye" is patched, the lazy eye must work more effectively with its partner. For some children, the squint may be so obvious that surgery is needed to bring the eyes into better alignment. The key to such problems is early referral to an ophthalmologist experienced in the care of children.

PARENT-TO-PARENT

"When my son Jonathan was born thirteen years ago, I had never heard the words *spina bifida*. When I was told of him having this birth defect, it was as though the whole world had stopped turning. I cannot begin to explain the deep hurt that I felt. I was so very scared. I felt that never again would I be able to smile or feel happiness in my life. My main concerns and worry were if I could take care of my son and meet his needs. I wondered if he would be happy and would have a fulfilling life. These were the questions that I kept asking myself. These feelings of despair engulfed me and were my thoughts every minute of the day.

When several surgeries and a long hospital stay were over, I was finally able to take my infant son home. Then something happened that took me by surprise. There were hours that went by and even days during which I wasn't constantly consumed with worry and hurt for my son.

Then the day came when he first smiled and my heart leaped with joy. I took great pride in his firsts: smiling, sitting alone, eating his first foods, and, of course, the day when he took his first steps. Yes, he took those steps with the aid of long leg braces and a walker, but I felt the joy and happiness of his accomplishments just I did with each of my other two children who do not have any disabilities. I then realized that I had a typical little boy with the same basic needs—love, encouragement, acceptance for what he can do, and understanding for what he cannot do.

I no longer worry if he will be happy, for he is. I no longer worry if my family will be happy, for we are. My life is no longer centered around his disability. It is just one part of him that we deal with and do the best we can."

"As a mother and father of a special three-year-old son born with spina bifida, some of the best advice we can offer is to have lots of patience and to try to instill confidence and independence in your child. We have tried our very best to encourage our son and to communicate that he *can* do anything he sets out to do. Most of all, we look to God for help, support, and strength in being the best parents possible for him."

"When our child was born with the birth defect spina bifida, we were unsure about his future. Mainly we were worried about his education. We didn't know if we could send him to day care, if he would attend school, or what level of education he would get. That big question was answered by the social worker in the clinic. We were informed about day care centers and development learning centers in our county that had trained people who work with special children like Brandon. From that advice, we got Brandon started in his education at four months old, and he is still learning and loves going to school. I really believe that all the special children can learn if we give them a chance."

"My wife and I just got tired of feeling like we had to face all these problems alone. That's when we decided to join a parents group at the day care center. We met other parents who were also struggling, and we were amazed to find out that we could offer them help and advice. Suddenly, it dawned on us that we weren't doing so badly and that we were getting back in control of our lives."

CHAPTER 7

Preschoolers

From three to five years of age are the magic years, marked by an incredible growth in language, imagination, and thought processes. New worlds open up in the minds of the preschooler, with new experiences, meanings, roles, games, and fears. It is a time of imaginary friends and real playmates, when a young child develops a sense of who she really is and how she should behave. Preschoolers begin to take the initiative in their relationships and in their play. They become more curious and more confident, learning to engage others and trying on new roles. These are rich years of great social and emotional growth. Those of us whose children have now grown beyond these magic years look back on these times—in photographs, videotapes, and memories—with great nostalgia!

In this chapter, I will describe some of the developmental issues that characterize these years. We will touch on the importance to a child with spina bifida of a developing sense of self and an awareness of the social world. Such key habilitation issues as the use of wheelchairs will be addressed, as will a few relevant medical issues, including latex allergy. I also provide some tips on how to prepare your child for surgery, as well as a few gems of advice from parents.

DEVELOPMENTAL ISSUES

Progressions and Expectations

It is often said that a child's development takes place not smoothly but in sudden spurts of growth followed by quiet periods or plateaus. The three-year-old child is typically poised for a dramatic spurt in receptive and expressive language. Vocabulary expands from perhaps one hundred words to several thousand during the preschool years! Expressive language progresses from simple labeling and requesting to a rich variety of sen-

Aspects of development	Three years	Four years	Five years
Adaptive	Imitates housework	Washes hands	Dresses independently
	Shows interest in toileting	Dresses self with assistance	
	Undresses	Helps with housework	
Fine-motor	Cuts with scissors	Can button	Tripod pencil grasp emerging
	Shows hand preference	Improved bimanual skills	Manages zippers
Language	Understands "in," "on," "under"	Understands "same," "different"	Names four colors
	Knows function of common object	Names one or two colors	Has emerging literacy skills
	Uses sentences of three to four words	Follows two-part commands	
	Mostly intelligible to strangers	Almost fully intelligible	
Cognitive	Copies circle	Copies cross	Copies square
	Can count three objects	Draws simple face	Understands number concepts
	Tells age and full name	Recognizes letters	Can count ten or more objects
			Draws face with body and limbs
			May write letters of alphabet
Personal-social	Growing sense of self	Imaginative play with friends	Recognizes own emotions
	Developing gender identity	Increasing independence	Learns more self-control

Figure 7.1. Developmental progressions in preschoolers, showing gains in adaptive, fine-motor, language, cognitive, and personal-social development

tences. Pronouns are used correctly, such prepositions as "in" and "under" emerge, and the functions of objects are described. These youngsters begin to use language to communicate how they feel—for example, "I'm tired" or "I'm hungry." Most four-year-olds know the basic colors and can name some animals. They can talk in complete sentences and engage others in conversation. By this age, speech should be almost completely intelligible to others. Figure 7.1 shows some of the developmental changes of the preschool years.

Preschool-age children also develop an interest in books and important skills that are precursors to literacy. They like to learn to recite the alphabet in song. They become fascinated with picture books that tell a story through a sequence of pictures. Some four- and five-year-olds will "read" picture books out loud, showing an appreciation of narrative and cause and effect, long before they have actually learned how to decode words.

Some toddlers with spina bifida seem precocious in their early language development. By the age of two years, they are reciting sentences and making conversation to the great delight of their parents. Such children learn the social value of language at an early age. They may have excellent verbal memory and perform well on certain preschool language measures. Although this strength in expressive language may not be matched by the child's development in other areas, such a profile has important implications for preschool education. Instead of focusing on areas of cognitive weakness, it is better to go with a young child's innate strengths in early education efforts.

The Growth of Imagination

Intimately linked with the spurt in language development is a period of dramatic growth in the mental processes that allow fantasy and imagination. Three- and four-year-olds develop the capacities to link events, to give meanings to observations, and to create solutions. This opens up a new world of magic and thought. Play becomes enriched by fantasy, and playmates are increasingly engaged in shared magical adventures. Many children have imaginary friends, who they know are not real in the sense that mommy and daddy and the cat are real but whom they will tell you about as if they were! An imaginary friend is not at all a sign of loneliness but a precious prize for a creative child. They are to be treasured!

The preschooler's thinking is typically egocentric. When asked, "Why does the sun shine?" a four-year-old may answer, "To keep me warm." Preschoolers may have a hard time understanding cause-and-effect relationships, instead invoking their own unique way of explaining and comprehending things. Because their thinking may not be constrained by the rational thought processes of their older siblings, they may have difficulty separating fact from fantasy. When they are prematurely exposed to frightening films and TV shows, their imaginations may get the better of them, leaving them terrified of animals, monsters, and ghosts and with assorted fears of the dark.

A Developing Sense of Self

These years are also marked by the development of a sense of "me" and, along with that, a great curiosity in others. The three-year-old develops an understanding of belonging in a family and likes to talk about mommy, daddy, brothers, sisters, and the dog. Within the family, there is a growing comprehension of roles and responsibilities, so that the four-year-old is interested in "how to behave" and responsive to limit setting and discipline. In the course of daily family life, the young child discovers a range of emotions within himself, learning self-control and acceptable ways to express these emotions. Growing cognitive abilities allow him then to replay events in his mind in "mental movies," helping him cope with these emotional surges and develop a clearer sense of who he is and how to behave.

Introduction to the Social World

Outside of the family, preschoolers start to make real connections with other children through play. With language and actions, they are able to communicate their fantasies and creative ideas, and they find that their play is enriched by the reciprocal input of others. Playmates learn from each other, infusing new twists, actions, and events into their games. In essence, they are experiencing each other through play and learning that two creative young minds are more fun than one! They imitate well and start to take on new roles. Some are real hams and love to try on these new identities, whereas others are a little shy. Preschoolers become increasingly aware of the responses they get from playmates and adults, and they learn from such feedback (some faster than others). As they see themselves reflected in the social world, they develop a clearer understanding of who they are.

It is so important for the young child with spina bifida to have opportunities to make these social connections. So many valuable social skills are learned through cooperative play. This fact seems so obvious to us now, yet it was not long ago that children with differences were excluded from the social mainstream. Many preschools were not prepared to deal with the challenges of including young children with physical disabilities. More than half the adolescents with spina bifida in our clinic have problems with social skills. I often wonder if these problems could have been prevented with good preschool education. I strongly recommend developmentally appropriate preschool education for all children with spina bifida. We will return to this issue in Chapter 11.

Boys and Girls: The Emergence of Sexual Identity

Also emerging in the three-year-old is a sense of gender identity. She may know she is a girl but not have much of an idea about what that means. Through an identification with her mother and great curiosity about sexual differences, that identification with being a girl grows. During these years, there may develop a particularly strong attachment between the boy and his mother or between the girl and her father.

This process of psychosexual development is wired into us, probably under genetic influences. It is just the same for children with and without spina bifida. A lack of genital sensation does not make a difference to the emergence of sexual identity. The only special consideration in preschoolers with spina bifida is that they may not encounter their own genitals as often in the course of self-exploration. Such self-exploration and sexual play are normal at this age. It may be helpful to show them different parts of their bodies, including their genitals, during bathing time or while playing in front of a mirror. It is good for them to know their bodies, and to do so contributes to their sense of self.

HABILITATION ISSUES

Dressing

Dressing is an important set of skills for a preschooler to learn. Those readers who have had to struggle to get the kids off to school in the morning will attest to this! The development of independent dressing skills follows a sequential pattern. Initially, a child learns to assist an adult by lifting arms, pushing hands into mittens, and so forth. Around two years of age, he usually learns how to remove simple items of clothing independently. Next, he figures out how to put on clothes, which may be quite a challenge, given that different kinds of clothing require completely different movements. Finally, by around age five or six, he learns some of the really tricky parts, such as fasteners, zippers, and shoelaces. Even when he has mastered all these skills, the whole process may take a long, long time, and in the ensuing years, these skills become increasingly efficient and automatic, eventually allowing him to get ready for school on time!

Dressing is a complex perceptual-motor task that requires the integration of a number of important functions. First, it entails body awareness—the appreciation of where one's body is in space and how its parts are related. Similarly, a child needs to have some spatial and perceptual ability to understand that a particular garment, such as a shirt, has a front and a back and that these features affect how the shirt should be put on. Second, dressing depends on motor planning, or the ability to plan a sequence of motor actions to accomplish a task. Third, it requires strength, coordination, adequate range of motion, and good hand function, especially. Fourth, sequential processing is important for a child to understand that, for example, underpants should go on before pants! Of course, independent dressing also requires the motivation to do the job by oneself.

Dressing can be a difficult challenge for the child with spina bifida for many reasons. Children with paraplegia tend to lack awareness of their legs. Weakness of certain muscle groups can make socks and pants hard to put on. For those youngsters with hand weakness or poor coordination and balance, the problems are compounded. Also, many children have difficulty with sequencing, needing assistance in doing the job in the right order.

In spite of these potential bumps in the road, kids with spina bifida can learn to dress themselves. It may take a long time, requiring patience from their parents. A tendency always exists to step in and take over the job for them, in the interests of time and sanity! But this tends to foster dependence, setting a precedent for other "help" that actually hinders self-help skills.

Here are a few tips that I have learned from parents. First, it is more helpful to have your child take over from you in completing the job than to have her start and then require you to finish it for her. When learning to put on a shirt, put it over the child's head and chest and then let her pull it all the way down and put her arms through the sleeves to complete the job. With a little practice, she can take over the step of pulling it over her head. Later still, she can add the previous step of actually getting the shirt in the right position to pull over her head. In other words, start at the end and work backward in steps (backward chaining). Oversized clothing is helpful, and it is a good idea to begin dressing programs at the beginning of summer, when fewer clothes must be put on. Also, remember to give lots of positive reinforcement along the way. Picture checklists can be helpful as prompts, assisting the child to do things in the required order (Figure 7.2).

Positioning is important. A child with poor trunk control may need special assistance such as sitting in her parent's lap or in a wheelchair so that support can be given to her abdomen while she puts on a shirt or her socks, for example. Sitting on the floor with her back up against a wall for support can also be helpful. When putting on pants, supine lying may be

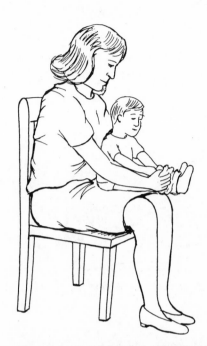

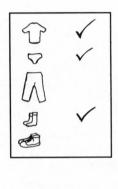

> **Dressing skills**
>
> Use appropriate positioning
> Practice in supported sit
> Hand-over-hand guidance
> Break task into steps
> Let child complete task
> Give praise and positive
>   reinforcement
> Use adaptive clothing

Figure 7.2. Helpful hints for dressing skills. A picture checklist helps a child accomplish this multistep task.

the most useful position, enabling some children to pull pants up all the way by lifting their buttocks sufficiently or rolling from side to side.

Additionally, adaptive clothing can be very useful. Baggy trousers are fashionable and can be large enough to fit comfortably over braces. Velcro fasteners allow many young kids to do for themselves. It is beneficial to get advice from an occupational therapist regarding positioning, techniques, and adaptive clothing. Several cottage industries produce clothing adaptive to different skill levels and to accommodate children who spend the day in wheelchairs. For example, such clothes may have a longer back seam so there's no gap, being shorter in the front to avoid bunching of the fabric. Pockets are also repositioned so they may be easily accessed without standing. Finding the manufacturers of adaptive clothing can be difficult, however, and the local chapter of the SBAA, the back pages of *Exceptional Parent* (a magazine for parents of children with disabilities), and word of mouth can lead you in the right direction.

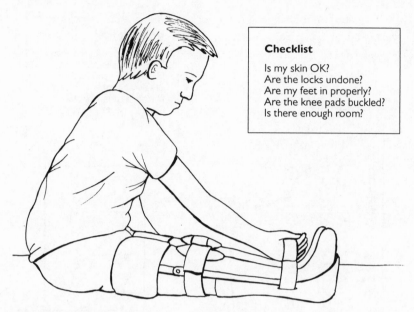

Checklist

Is my skin OK?
Are the locks undone?
Are my feet in properly?
Are the knee pads buckled?
Is there enough room?

Figure 7.3. Teaching a child how to put on braces, and a mental checklist to ensure safety

Other Activities of Daily Living

There are many opportunities for children with spina bifida to assist in self-care. Last week 1 saw a ten-year-old boy who was dependent on his mother or father to change his diaper properly. He had the requisite skills to do so, but they had always done it for him. During the same clinic, I saw a three-year-old boy who was able to undo the tabs, take off the old diaper, pull up the new one, and fasten the tabs. His parents had enlisted his help in diaper changes for about a year, and he understood that they valued his independent contribution! Of course, different children have different capabilities and cannot all be expected to accomplish the same self-help tasks. Each child should be encouraged from a very early age to do what he or she is capable of doing.

Similarly, the skills involved in taking braces on and off should be actively taught. Preschoolers can learn to undo fastenings, lift their legs up, and remove the braces. Putting the braces on is a little more challenging, and physical therapists will provide valuable advice. Generally, one should start with the feet and work upward (Figure 7.3). Even three-year-old children should be able to assist to varying degrees by positioning their legs and by fastening and securing the locks. Marking the position of the big toe on a pair of AFOs may help a young child identify which AFO goes on the left leg and which on the right.

Bathing is another area of daily living that provides an opportunity for self-care and self-exploration while having fun. The use of nonslip surfaces is very helpful for the young child who is still struggling with postural control. Positioning may be enhanced by using a little tub seat or an inflatable inner tube. Older children may find it helpful to use a grab bar to help them get down into the bathtub and pull themselves out. Many children prefer to sit on a shower bench if the transfer in and out of the bathtub is very difficult. It is important to safeguard against injuries from falling on a hard surface without protective bracing. In addition, I have seen a few kids with severe scalds from very hot water. Water heaters should be set at around 125 degrees, and the water temperature should always be carefully tested before the child places his or her foot in the tub.

Wheelchairs, Transfers, and Independence

Although a sturdy stroller may be ideal for the toddler, most children with spina bifida who are not able to walk as their usual means of mobility need a wheelchair by the time they are three or four years old. Figure 7.4 shows a typical modern wheelchair and its parts. Wheelchairs are manufactured by many companies and are advertised extensively in magazines such as *Exceptional Parent*. Information can also be obtained from your physical therapist, orthotics department (brace shop), and local health care equipment supply companies.

In selection of the appropriate wheelchair, seating position is extremely important. The chair should provide the proper fit and proper support. The seat should be wide enough to accommodate the child comfortably, without confining the child, limiting adjustments of posture, or interfering with transfers. There should certainly be a space of at least one inch between the child's hips and the arms of the chair. If the seat is too wide, however, the chair may be hard for the child to propel, and it may not provide adequate postural support, especially for children with thoracic spina bifida. For ideal support and to avoid the development of pressure areas, children with a spinal deformity may need specially made seat inserts.

Equally important is the footrest height. The child should be able to sit comfortably with his weight evenly supported along the length of his thighs and with approximately ninety degrees of flexion at hips, knees, and ankles. If the footrests are too low, his feet will dangle, and there will

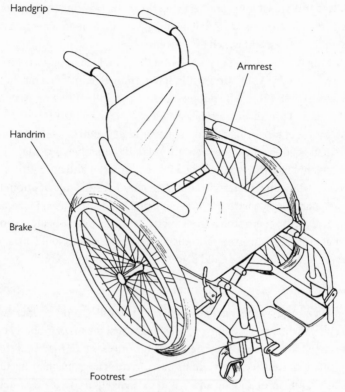

Handgrip

Armrest

Handrim

Brake

Footrest

Figure 7.4. The anatomy of a wheelchair

be excessive pressure on the backs of the thighs from the front edge of the seat. If they are too high, there will be excessive flexion and too much weight on his buttocks.

In addition to these considerations, the seat length should be long enough to provide support for the thighs, but not so long that the edge of the seat puts pressure on the calves. For a good fit, there should be a gap of at least one inch between the front edge of the seat and the top of the calves.

With all the styles and options to choose from, arriving at a decision regarding a wheelchair can be overwhelming. It is advisable to have an expert physician prescribe the chair, with input from a physical therapist and/or occupational therapist regarding the individual needs of the child.

As in other aspects of self-care, children must be instructed in the safe use of the chair. They need to know that the seat belt must be securely fastened and worn consistently. They must use both brakes to lock the wheels when the chair is stationary or for transfers. They need to check

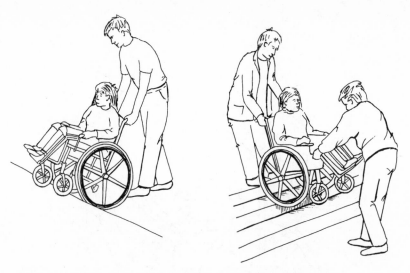

Figure 7.5. The correct use of a wheelchair on stairs and curbs

the position of their feet on the footrests. Children must even know how to fall safely and, having fallen, how to get back into the chair from the ground. Having worked as the doctor at a spina bifida camp and witnessed kids zooming down hills at breakneck speed, I suggest they learn to exercise some caution!

Parents, teachers, and other care providers must also know some wheelchair basics, including the use of the tipping lever when mounting curbs or traveling on rough terrain. Although communities are increasingly accessible to wheelchairs, at times it will be necessary to pull the wheelchair up steps backward or to maneuver downstairs (Figure 7.5).

Transfers require complex sequences of movements on the part of young children and their care providers. If done correctly, they can be efficient and safe. If done inexpertly, they can be exhausting and also lead to injury, for both the child and the adult. For young children, the simplest means of transfer is to lift and carry. Once the wheelchair is in a suitable position, the wheels should be locked, and the adult should position himself or herself right up against the chair. For the preschooler, a one-person lift is usually easily accomplished by holding the child with one arm around the back and the other under the legs. For older and heavier children, it may be necessary to use the two-person lift, in which one adult takes the legs and the other adult takes the child under the arms and across the chest from behind (Figure 7.6). No matter which method, it is essential to use the legs to lift, not the back. By keeping the back straight

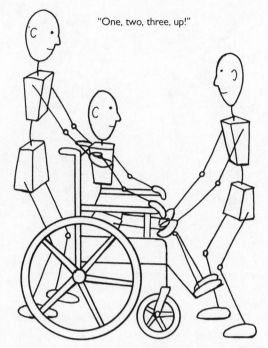

"One, two, three, up!"

Figure 7.6. The two-person lift: adults should have
straight backs and bent knees.

and avoiding twisting movements, it is possible to escape back injuries
and slipped disks.

There are other transfers that require more active participation on the
part of the preschooler. How much of the transfer the child can accomplish independently depends on his or her sitting balance, strength, cognitive abilities, and motivation to succeed. It is important that adults
allow the child to participate, at the same time ensuring that the transfer is safe. Sliding board transfers enable the young child to move from
the wheelchair to the bed, to another chair, or into a car, by moving in
the sitting position along a smooth wooden board. It requires good trunk
control and sitting balance, as well as considerable upper body strength.
When transferring from the wheelchair, the chair should be locked, with
the armrest and legrest on the one side removed. The stand-pivot transfer
is useful for a child who can support some weight with his or her legs. If
transferring to the toilet, for example, the wheelchair is maneuvered close
to the toilet and locked. The legrests are removed, and the feet are positioned on the floor. The child pushes up to standing, using the armrests
of the wheelchair, and then moves one hand to the grab bar by the toilet.

By pivoting the body, the child is able to get into position to gently lower himself or herself down into sitting.

There are other ways of transferring that are safe and effective. It is important to ask the physical therapist for advice and to work on these skills consistently. As in all aspects of living with a disability, a positive, can-do attitude and creative troubleshooting go a long way toward solving the problems of self-help skills.

Promoting Ambulation

Those preschoolers who are ambulatory will become more proficient in walking during these years. Many will spontaneously progress from a slow four-point gait to a smooth and coordinated two-point gait, in which one crutch moves forward at the same time as the opposite leg. The use of games can help a child to develop ambulatory skills and confidence, as well as enhancing safety. Modified baseball, in which the child uses a crutch as a bat while maintaining balance with the other crutch, is one such enjoyable activity. Adaptive playgrounds have been built in many communities and are well worth the investment, allowing disabled young children to explore the limits of their physical abilities safely. For those children who are fearful and have obvious balance problems, it may be beneficial to engage the assistance of a physical therapist to work on gait training while improving balance and movement patterns. It may also be helpful to teach these children how to fall safely, so they feel less afraid when walking in their braces.

Fine-Motor Function

At least two-thirds of children with spina bifida have significant delays on a variety of measures of fine-motor function. Delay in fine-motor function may affect the child's ability to master self-help skills, especially dressing. School readiness skills are also affected by these difficulties. Pencil control, cutting, and coloring are often elusive. Eye-hand coordination is characteristically poor; thus ball skills, block construction skills, and other common preschool activities are usually below average. I have seen a few youngsters with spina bifida who have great difficulty getting their eyes to focus on what they are trying to accomplish with their hands. Their gaze tends to wander off, so that they are without the important visual feedback that they need to accomplish a given task.

Fine-motor delays are due to underlying differences in neurologic function, including the cerebellar and midbrain structures that are involved in the Chiari malformation. In addition, there is evidence that myelination of central white matter structures is somewhat delayed in children with spina bifida, which probably also has an impact on fine-motor speed, coordination, and dexterity.

Figure copying and drawing skills are also delayed. Using a common assessment tool such as the Beery Test of Visual Motor Integration (VMI), more than half of all children with spina bifida are below the average range. Their drawings are often poorly organized, and pencil control is problematic. These concerns are more evident in those who have hydrocephalus than in those who do not. As these children progress in the early elementary grades, fine-motor problems are seen in their handwriting difficulties. I will discuss these issues in the next chapter.

The first step toward helping children overcome or bypass these difficulties is a thorough assessment by an expert. Most occupational therapists are very experienced in determining the nature of the problem. Some children have significant motor planning problems (dyspraxia), struggling to put together a plan for a sequence of motor actions. Others have difficulties with motor implementation: their movements are appropriately sequenced but are poorly regulated, clumsy, and inefficient. Many children lack adequate feedback from their muscles and joints (finger agnosia) and therefore are overly reliant on visual monitoring and feedback. They typically hold their crayons and pencils in a very fisted grasp, which does not permit movement of the small joints of the hand. Instead, they have to move the wrist and forearm, a pattern of movement that increases writing fatigue and prevents the development of fluidity in handwriting. They also tend to have their eyes very close to the page as they carefully oversee the movements of their hands. Some typical patterns of fine-motor dysfunction are shown in Figure 7.7.

There are many options for therapy, the choice of which will be guided by the child's age and capabilities and by the nature of his fine-motor dysfunction. The occupational therapist may work on obtaining the optimal seating position, in which the young child is well supported and the arms and hands are maximally freed to move. The use of such adaptive equipment as desk easels or cutout tables can be helpful in this regard. If there are significant motor planning problems, the therapist may use sensory integration techniques to help the child establish new motor sequences. Children with finger agnosia may also benefit from these approaches and from the utilization of different textures and materials for manipulation.

Specific toys and adaptive equipment may enhance the child's skills. For the child approaching kindergarten, the use of adaptive pencil grips

	Dyspraxia	"Clumsiness"	Finger agnosia	Eye-hand incoordination
Nature of problem	Motor planning	Efficiency	Feedback regulation	Visual-motor integration
Typical difficulties	Initiating movements	Spilling things	Close visual monitoring	Catching
	Imitating gestures	Overshooting	Poor automatization	Cutting
	Putting items in the wrong order	Using excessive force	Fisted, tight pencil grip	Coloring
		Using too many muscle groups		

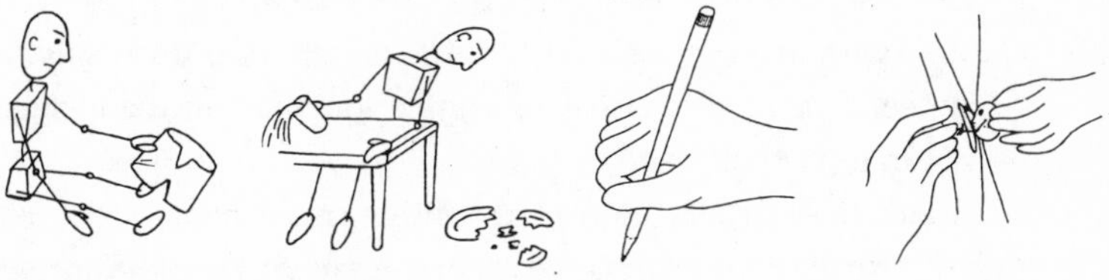

Figure 7.7. Common patterns of fine-motor dysfunction

may promote the appropriate tripod grasp. As in all things, children improve with practice, and the job of the therapist is to make therapy fun, keeping children coming back for more. It should also be stressed that the more severe problems are unlikely to be cured, although treatment can still be beneficial.

Visual-Perceptual Function

Developmental functions are often closely associated in the brain, and therefore it is unusual to find a child with just one discrete yet significant area of dysfunction. Two very closely associated functions are fine-motor function and visual-perceptual function. So it is that a large proportion, around 50 percent, of children with spina bifida perform poorly on tasks of visual-perceptual function. Although their eyes may have normal acuity (an assumption that needs to be checked, as mentioned in the last chapter), they have trouble processing and interpreting the visual information that they receive. It is analogous to the child with normal hearing who has language-processing problems. The circuits for processing visual information are complex and involve different areas of the brain. It appears that the brain differences associated with spina bifida disrupt the normal development of some of these circuits. It is not purely an effect of hydrocephalus, because similar patterns of dysfunction are seen in many children with spina bifida but without hydrocephalus.

Visual-perceptual dysfunction may take many forms. Some children have the greatest difficulty sustaining visual attention. They may be able to focus attention quite well with auditory input, but when the information is visual, they have trouble picking out salient details, their gaze shifting to other things. They tend to examine the stimulus superficially as a gestalt and may be unable to examine the details within the stimulus. When confronted with an array of choices, they often fail to scan the choices systematically, instead responding impulsively by choosing the first one they see or becoming distracted from the task altogether. For children with such problems, the typical preschool and kindergarten class worksheets that involve visual discrimination, matching, and attention to detail can be very difficult.

Related to visual attention is the ability to make figure-ground determinations—to sort out what is the essential, salient visual information and what is the background. The reader is probably familiar with examples of ambiguous figure-ground, in which a picture appears one way if one focuses on certain elements, but another way if one makes subtle shifts of attention. Of course, most often we are not presented with such ambiguous information in our day-to-day lives, and we can pick out the striking aspects of form quite easily and automatically to make sense of the information we get through our eyes. For many children with spina bifida, this process is not so automatic, and they encounter ambiguity quite frequently. Consequently, they may have trouble "seeing the forest for the trees."

Another related phenomenon is the appreciation of spatial relationships—that is, how objects are related to one another in space. Many children with spina bifida are confused about spatial relationships. They may struggle with concepts of "above and below" and "left and right," and they may have difficulty following instructions that involve such spatial relationships. They may show weaknesses in depth perception and understanding of form constancy (how a thing can look different from different angles). These differences in spatial relationships are sometimes reflected in their drawings. In examining the "people drawings" created by children with spina bifida, I have seen some characteristic features of their drawings of themselves (Figure 7.8). They often portray disconnected limbs or a single limb projecting from their bodies, an expression of their individual and unique visual-perceptual experience.

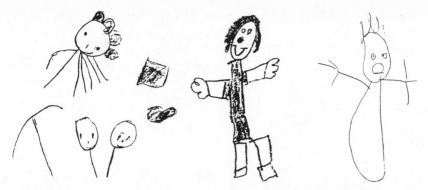

Figure 7.8. Examples of drawings by children with spina bifida. Notice the disorganization, perceptual problems, and single or absent lower limbs.

Perhaps the first step in management is to ensure that the child has adequate vision. Acuity and binocular vision should be checked by an experienced ophthalmologist. Intervention and educational strategies for visual-perceptual problems are included in Chapter 11.

MEDICAL ISSUES

A variety of orthopedic problems of the knees, ankles, and feet may arise throughout childhood, including during these preschool years. For convenience, I will discuss some of these problems and their management in this chapter.

Knees and Ankles

The stability of the knee joint depends on the balanced functioning of the two main groups of muscles that act on the knee: the quadriceps (quads) in front, and the hamstrings behind (Figure 7.9). If the quadriceps are nonfunctioning, such as in thoracic or high-lumbar lesions, the knee joint is likely to be lax. Increased tone in one of the muscle groups can lead to the development of contractures—for example, hamstrings that are overactive will lead to flexion contractures of the knees. This presents a problem to the ambulatory child, who needs to have a straight leg to walk with a relatively efficient gait. Flexion contractures of this sort are usually treated with soft tissue releases and/or hamstring releases, in addition to physical therapy (Figure 7.10).

Some children have overactive quads relative to hamstrings; thus they develop extension contractures and have very limited flexion at the knee

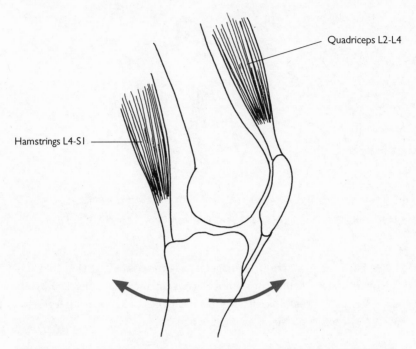

Figure 7.9. Muscle balance around the knee joint. The hamstrings flex (bend) the knee, and the quadriceps extend (straighten) it.

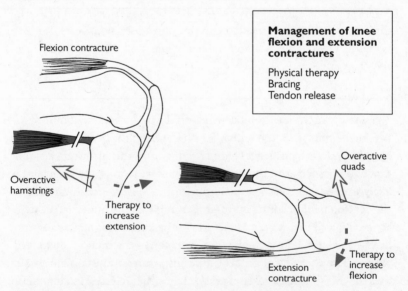

Figure 7.10. The management of knee flexion and extension contractures. In addition to physical therapy and bracing, surgical release of tendons may be necessary to restore a more normal position.

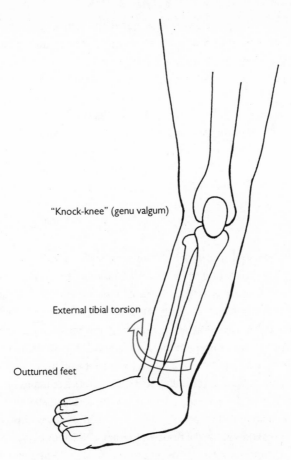

"Knock-knee" (genu valgum)

External tibial torsion

Outturned feet

Figure 7.11. External tibial torsion and genu valgum (knock-knee). The muscle imbalance in the lower leg leads to outward turning of the feet.

joints. This can be a problem for wheelchair seating, because the child's legs would project forward and the feet would not rest comfortably on the footrests. Such problems can usually be prevented by physical therapy and bracing but may also require surgical release.

Another common problem is tibial torsion, or twisting of the tibia (the main bone in the lower leg). Many children with midlevel-lumbar spina bifida develop external tibial torsion, associated with genu valgum (knock-knee). As a result, the lower leg tends to be angled outward, and the foot is positioned so that the feet point out. These problems are most evident when the child is walking, and they can become increasingly obvious to the observer as the child grows older (Figure 7.11). For the young child, the Denis-Browne splint can be worn at night to maintain the feet in a neutral position and to counteract the tendency to go into external rotation. For the older child, the use of orthoses to provide stability around the knee joint and to maintain appropriate alignment during walking is essential.

It is important to assess and record the alignment of the knees, ankles, and feet each time the child is seen in the clinic for comprehensive care. Significant changes in positioning, tone, and posture may indicate tethering of the spine, cord syrinx, or other such neurologic complications. Early detection of these problems may allow for more effective management and prevention of further disability.

Foot Problems

Half of all babies with spina bifida are born with a significant foot deformity. This may affect one or both feet and may not be symmetrical. This congenital deformity is a result of muscle weakness, which leads to abnormal positioning in the uterus. During early childhood, the postural effects of gravity, as well as weight bearing and growth, can lead to further deformity. The consequences of such deformity are twofold. First, for children who are ambulatory, a plantigrade foot in neutral position (that is, a foot whose sole is oriented to strike the ground squarely) is essential for optimal walking. Second, a well-positioned foot distributes pressure evenly over a large surface and is therefore less likely to run into problems from skin breakdown. Even a nonambulatory child should have appropriate management of foot deformities to prevent skin breakdown. Different typical appearances of foot deformities are shown in Figure 7.12.

In mild cases the equinus deformity or equinovarus deformity can be treated by manipulations and casting, but most need subcutaneous release of the Achilles tendon with postoperative splinting. Such operations are easily done as outpatient procedures. Clubfoot deformities may be manageable by manipulations and casting but also require soft tissue releases. For severe and rigid deformities, talectomy (the removal of the talus bone) is necessary. Calcaneovalgus deformities occur mainly in low-lumbar spina bifida, as a result of strong anterior tibials and absent or weak gastrocnemius and soleus muscles. Although physical therapy designed to stretch out the contractures and appropriate bracing may be sufficient, some children need a tibialis anterior tendon transfer to enable the active muscle to exert a more balanced force around the ankle joint. Cavus deformities may tend to increase during childhood, possibly requiring plantar release surgery eventually. Vertical talus (rigid, rocker-bottom feet) is a deformity that

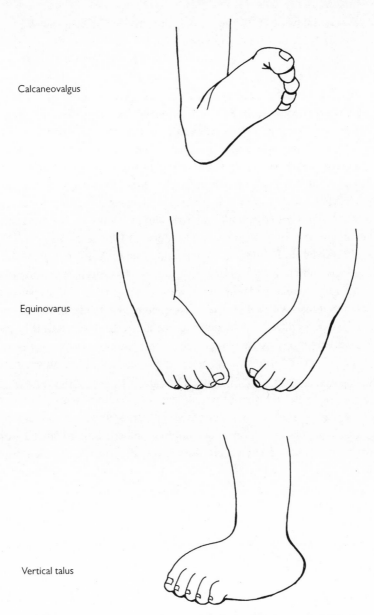

Calcaneovalgus

Equinovarus

Vertical talus

Figure 7.12. Typical appearances of foot deformities in spina bifida

usually cannot be dealt with by casting and may require surgical release of the contracted ligaments and tendons.

Warning: Allergic to Latex!

During recent years, there has been increasing recognition of the high incidence of allergy to latex among children with spina bifida. The unfolding of this saga began in the late 1980s, when anesthesiologists encountered a few sporadic cases of anaphylaxis (severe allergic reaction) during surgery. In 1989, two such cases of intraoperative anaphylaxis in children with myelomeningocele were reported. The following year, anesthesiologists in Milwaukee examined a cluster of such cases and realized that ten out of the eleven had spina bifida (the eleventh case had a congenital bladder abnormality). In 1991, the Centers for Disease Control investigated this new clinical problem, confirming that the cause was indeed an allergic reaction to latex and that the problem was especially common in children with spina bifida. In fact, it was estimated that 18 to 40 percent of all individuals with spina bifida were allergic to latex. Since than, clinics such as ours have been scrambling to educate families about this risk and to take appropriate steps to prevent clinical problems from arising.

Latex is derived from the rubber tree, *Hevea brasiliensis*, cultivated in many parts of the world, including Malaysia. The tree produces a sticky sap that is combined with other chemicals to produce latex. The latex is widely used in hospitals, especially in operating rooms: masks, gloves, tape, tourniquets, and other intravenous equipment contain latex. Latex urinary and enema catheters are used frequently. Feeding nipples, dental dams, condoms, and diaphragms may also contain latex. The catheters commonly used for intermittent catheterization are synthetic and do not contain latex. In fact, half of so-called rubber products are latex free. The problem is that latex is a common ingredient of a number of nonmedical items with which children are likely to come into contact. For example, balloons, Koosh balls, rubber bands, and other toys may set off allergic reactions. Of these, balloons are the most common. Many parents report that their child developed facial redness, itching, and puffiness after blowing up a balloon at a birthday party. There is even some cross-reactivity with certain foods, such as avocado. One of the most dramatic accidental exposures occurred recently at a spina bifida camp, when some experts in bass fishing came to the camp to show the kids how to catch bass in the lake. Although the kids fished with live crickets, they were each given a little bag of rubber worms to take home with them. As soon as we realized this, we energetically rounded up a few hundred of these things before

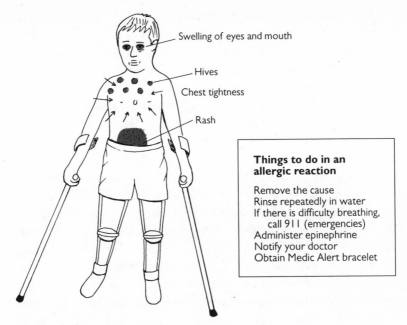

Swelling of eyes and mouth

Hives

Chest tightness

Rash

Things to do in an allergic reaction

Remove the cause
Rinse repeatedly in water
If there is difficulty breathing,
    call 911 (emergencies)
Administer epinephrine
Notify your doctor
Obtain Medic Alert bracelet

Figure 7.13. Symptoms and signs of latex allergy, with things to do in the event of an allergic reaction

anybody developed allergic symptoms! The point is that we all need to be vigilant about this problem.

The symptoms and signs of latex allergy are shown in Figure 7.13. Of course, not every child with spina bifida has latex allergy. It is more common in those who have a history of allergies and asthma. It is also more likely to develop in those who have had multiple operations, because surgery is generally associated with major exposure to latex. Also, older children are more likely to run into problems than are younger ones. Unfortunately, no good test exists for latex allergies. Obviously, if a child has a history of allergic symptoms associated with exposure to latex, he or she should be considered latex allergic. I think young children with a tendency to develop allergic symptoms and asthma should also be presumed to be allergic to latex. For those without such a history, it may be helpful to do latex skin testing (prick test, not intradermal test), although this can precipitate a major allergic reaction in a sensitive individual. Some people recommend a blood test called RAST (radioallergosorbent test), but the test is not very sensitive. Indeed, the current recommendation of the Nursing Council of the Spina Bifida Association of America is that everybody with spina bifida should be on latex precautions.

In the event of an allergic reaction, the exposure material should be removed, and the exposed area should be washed immediately. For mild symptoms that are not progressive, a dose of an antihistamine may be sufficient. For more severe symptoms, Emergency Medical Services should be notified immediately. The rapid administration of epinephrine can be lifesaving in cases of anaphylaxis, and highly sensitive individuals may do well to carry self-injectable epinephrine in case of emergency. Those who are latex allergic should also wear Medic Alert bracelets.

The mainstay of management, however, is the avoidance of exposure in medical and other settings. Vinyl gloves, silk tape, plastic/vinyl/silicone catheters, and other nonlatex substitutes can and should be used routinely in the health care of children with spina bifida. Precautions should be taken especially in operating rooms and dental offices, where exposure can be sudden and enormous. I have included a list of latex-containing products and potential substitutes that was produced by the SBAA in December 1993 (Figure 7.14). A cautious approach is justified in clinical decision making regarding latex allergy in spina bifida.

EMOTIONAL ISSUES

Preparing Your Child for Hospitalization

Leaving the safety and familiarity of home and entering the strange and threatening world of the hospital, with its many uniformed strangers, unfamiliar noises, and unexpected, painful experiences, is among the most stressful experiences a young child can have. Although pediatric wards and hospitals are much more child centered than they used to be, child patients inevitably feel vulnerable and fearful. How they cope depends on a number of factors, including the child's age, stage of development, personality and temperament, familiarity with the hospital and staff, the presence and support of the parents, and the degree of pain and discomfort. For many two- and three-year-old children, the overriding concern is, "Will mommy come back?" Assurances that a parent will return soon mean little to an anxious child with no sense of time. Sleep disturbances, loss of appetite, temper tantrums, and listlessness are common behavioral responses of the toddler. The preschooler may cope with the stress of hospitalization differently, using imagination and magical thinking to explain and understand his or her experiences and perhaps tolerating separation from parents more easily because he or she now understands that out of sight is not out of mind. At this age children may easily misconstrue events, developing fantasies about why they are in hospital or how

Products that may contain latex	Some latex-free alternatives
Art supplies—paint, markers, glue	
Balloons	Mylar balloons
Balls—Koosh balls, tennis balls	Thornton sports ball (vinyl)
Carpet backing, gym floors	
Chewing gum	
Condoms, diaphragms	Condoms made of polyurethane or tachylon
	Natural-skin condoms
Crutches—axillary and hand pads	Cover with stockinette
Disposable diapers	Huggies
Elastic on legs and waists of clothing	
Feeding nipples	Silicone nipples
Foam rubber lining of braces	Line with cloth or felt
Gloves for cleaning or use in the kitchen	Vinyl gloves, cotton liners
Pacifiers	Plastic, silicone, or vinyl pacifiers
Toys—rubber ducky, teething toys	Plastic, cloth, and vinyl toys
Racquet and tool handles	Vinyl and leather handles
Raincoats, rubber boots	Plastic or vinyl
Rubber bands	String
Rubber pants (diapers)	Cloth, Velcro closures
Water toys, swim/scuba equipment	Plastic or vinyl toys
Wheelchair cushions, tires	Neoprene cushions or fabric-covered seat
	Use leather gloves
Zippered plastic storage bags	Waxed paper, plain plastic bags

Figure 7.14. Latex-containing products and potential substitutes. This list is published with the permission of the Spina Bifida Association of America as a guide for families but will change as we learn more about latex allergy and as manufacturers improve their products.

they may have caused the hospitalization to occur. No matter how often the "facts" are presented, a child may go on believing his or her own ego-centric explanations.

Children commonly respond to hospitalizations with temporary regressions in their development. Such regressions possibly represent adaptive and protective responses of the child to the new, stressful situation. Protests, tantrums, and withdrawal may serve to protect the child emotionally, to elicit help and caring from others, and to defend against the perceived loss of a parent. Parents should anticipate such responses and understand their significance.

There are many strategies that can help prepare a child for surgery or hospitalization. For elective procedures, it is important to provide a simple description. Toys and coloring books may be useful, and a visit to the hospital to acquaint parents and children to the new setting often helps them feel more at ease. For the preschooler and early-school-age child, it is a good idea to explore the child's concepts of her or his illness and the reasons for the hospitalization. Misconceptions can be addressed, reassurances provided, and concerns discussed.

While your child is in hospital, it is important to be truthful about procedures. Age-appropriate descriptions prepare children and enable them to cope more easily. Children should be allowed to participate in their medical care to feel that they have some control over their bodies, even during hospitalization and illness. Offering choices, allowing them to perform "procedures" on dolls in play therapy, and letting them handle medical equipment can be beneficial in this regard.

Ideally, hospitalizations should be avoided! Unfortunately, in the life of a child with a chronic illness such as spina bifida, hospitalizations are to be expected. A successful hospitalization is one in which healing takes place, both physical and psychological. Parents should emerge from the experience with a deeper understanding of their children and an enhanced sense of competency as guardians of their children's health. Children should emerge from a period of hospitalization with improved health, as well as enhancement in their ability to deal ably with adverse, stressful experiences.

PARENT-TO-PARENT

"Those preschool years were the most frustrating but also the most exciting. Every day, we would overcome some barrier or see a little improvement in Jason's skills. And then just when you think you're really getting somewhere, suddenly there's a new obstacle."

"My friends would tell me how strong I was to be able to handle it all so well. Mostly, I was just trying to keep from going under. . . . I didn't feel like such a strong person. But then I would sometimes stop and look back at what we had accomplished and feel just a little proud. I think that these challenges help us parents to feel stronger and more confident."

"I guess the thing that has helped the most is to look on the bright side. For some people the glass looks half empty, but to me it's half full most of the time. There are a lot of problems, but you have to take them on with a positive attitude. My husband and I didn't dwell on the big questions that are there in the back of our minds. We just tried to move ahead, one small step at a time, one little day at a time."

"One of the hardest things for me was going back to work, but it was the best decision in the long run. Jessica was my whole world. I was hardly going out at all, not even seeing my friends, and I was getting depressed. My husband and the doctor were telling me to put her in preschool, but I resisted. I thought that she was too little and frail to go somewhere without me! But then I got talking to other parents in the clinic, and I could see that it would be in Jessica's best interests to get her started in preschool. I never figured how helpful going back to work would be for me. It got me out the house, meeting other people, and doing something else that I could be satisfied with."

"Having a child with spina bifida doesn't make your marriage fall apart. But not dealing with your feelings sure can. I was angry, confused, and becoming more and more distant. My wife had all the responsibility with Justin and the other kids. I felt disconnected from the family and spent more and more time at work. Finally, we reached breaking point, and she spelled it out for me: either I got involved and started to share in family life, or I got out! We've been through a lot, but we feel like we have a richer relationship now than ever before."

The School-Age Child

Middle childhood, spanning the years from age six through age twelve, is a period in which children learn the skills that will be essential to their later survival. They learn about their culture and what will be expected of them. Most important, they learn to be productive citizens. Whereas play is at the heart of the preschool years, work is at the heart of middle childhood. This work should not be grueling or unpleasant but fun to do and satisfying to accomplish. Indeed, for a child engrossed in collecting rocks or drawing horses, work and play become the same thing. Children learn the value of working to meet goals and master challenges.

Nowhere is this more evident than in school. School is the arena of success and failure in middle childhood. Each day at school, the child has to cope with challenges. For many, the classroom is the most challenging environment, one where increasingly complex tasks are presented. For others, the playground and lunchroom are the most difficult and harrowing places, fraught with their own complex social hazards. It is no wonder that many children come home from school like knights from battle, somewhat bruised, tarnished, and irritable! But with each new challenge they confront and with each task they master, there comes a growing sense of competence. Erikson wrote of this stage as one of "industry versus inferiority," from which children should emerge with a stronger identity, a knowledge of their strengths and weaknesses, and a belief in the value and the fun of work.

In this chapter, I discuss how having a chronic illness in general and having spina bifida in particular affects middle childhood development. I shall address learning and learning disabilities, attention deficit, and other school-related problems that may occur, as well as management of these problems. I then present some habilitation issues, especially those of continence. Details about clean intermittent catheterization and bowel programs will be provided. Among the medical issues, I will cover growth, precocious puberty, urinary tract infections, scoliosis, tethering, and seizures. We shall also examine some emotional issues that may occur in middle childhood.

DEVELOPMENTAL ISSUES

Progressions and Expectations

The years of middle childhood are characterized by dramatic increases in demands and expectations, some of which are shown in Figure 8.1. School-age children make major strides toward independence and self-reliance. As friends and the peer group become increasingly important, children begin the process of separation that gathers steam during adolescence—sleepovers and overnight camps are a milestone in this progression. The situation is compounded by the presence of a chronic illness or condition such as spina bifida, which imposes additional demands and places obstacles in the way of a child making these tentative steps to independence. Moreover, negotiating the tightrope that parents walk in their efforts to allow this progression while still providing protection and support is even harder for parents of children with a chronic illness.

The brain is about 90 percent of its adult size by the time a child is five years old. Nevertheless, the additional neurologic development that takes place between the ages of six and twelve is remarkable to observe! Children progress from the magical thinking of the preschool years to concrete operations. New concepts become apparent to them, and they develop the cognitive ability to engage in such mental operations as addition and subtraction. They learn to complete complex, multistep procedures. Serial order and the preservation of sequences become increasingly important in their thinking.

The most important of these cognitive developments is the ability to use symbols, such as letters and numerals. Children decode and encode information using these symbols, with reading and performing simple arithmetic serving as a gateway to a world of learning. Children vary greatly in their readiness to pass through this gateway.

At the same time, there is a dawning of the capacity to reason, to consider more than one aspect of a problem as the child seeks a solution. For some, problem-solving abilities develop easily, whereas others need greater assistance to find and use strategies. As the child gains these abilities to reflect and evaluate, there develops the capacity to evaluate one's abilities and products in comparison with one's peers. Whereas six-year-

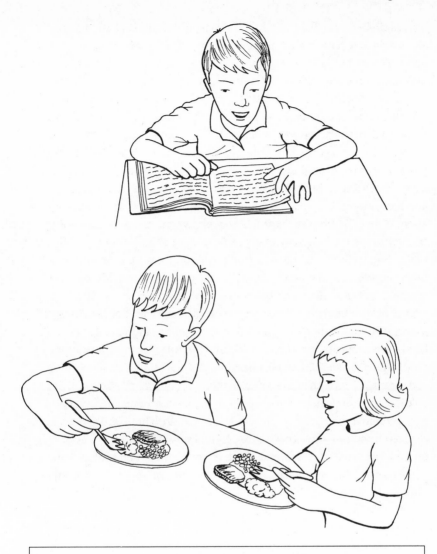

Cognitive	Language	Personal-social
Conservation of matter	Written language	Reflection and insight
Mental operations	Social use of language	Self-knowledge
Multistep procedures	Appreciation of grammar	Rules and schedules
Sequential processing	and syntax	Delay of gratification
Problem solving	Narrative organization	Development of
Increasing attention focus	Vocabulary development	conscience
	Understanding of humor	Control of impulses
	and ambiguity	

Figure 8.1. Some of the changing demands and expectations in middle childhood. Cognitive, language, and personal-social skills develop rapidly during these years.

old children do not have much of a concept of individual ability, most eight-year-olds have a growing sense of how they measure up to their peers. These years are marked by the development of insight and self-knowledge, a process that really matures in adolescence. The implications for a child with differences is that this period marks their first real understanding of being different. This realization, although sometimes painful, is essential for the development of a child with spina bifida.

The school years impose another set of demands on children that some find very hard to meet. Suddenly, children have to make a transition from the freewheeling preschool world of play to the rigors of schedules, rules, and regulations. They have to stand in line, wait their turn, and delay gratification. Children are expected to comply with these demands, and those who are not developmentally ready to make this transition are often called "immature." The increasing emphasis on rules leads to a growing internalization of rules and a respect for authority. These years mark the emergence of conscience and the growth of a sense of morality.

It is no wonder that the school-age child sometimes needs to escape from the harsh realities and imposed order of school and schoolwork and let his or her imagination run free! A healthy indulgence in fantasy is typical of these years and may take many forms. Some may get hooked on video games, losing their identities as they shoot down aliens or leap for golden rings! Some identify strongly with heroes, real or imaginary. Sports stars and movie characters capture children's imaginations and give them opportunities to channel their aggressive and sexual impulses in ways that do no harm. Like anything else, these pursuits can get out of hand and detract form other valuable pastimes, but for the vast majority of kids, it's just part of growing up.

The overriding imperative for school-age children is the quest for social acceptance. Once children have formed primary relationships within the family, they begin to establish social ties with their peers. By the age of ten to twelve years, the search for friendship and popularity and avoidance of humiliation at all costs become relentless campaigns, which may well take precedence over academic stardom or pleasing parents. Children feel enormous pressure to define themselves by being like others their age, and the drive toward conformity becomes a nearly tyrannical force. Certain settings, like the bus, the cafeteria, and the gymnasium, provide the backdrop for fierce and telling social transactions. Being labeled or called names is an ever present threat.

Researchers have studied popularity and unpopularity in school-age children, identifying four groups of children: popular children are acceptable, sought after and respected by their peers; controversial children are highly liked by some and highly disliked by others; neglected children are relatively inconspicuous, and few children seem to know them very well; and rejected children are ostracized from the peer group. To a large extent, a child's peer status is determined by her or his social skills. Popular children are skillful at entering a social situation or a conversation. They are responsive to their peers, knowing how to make them feel wanted, recognized, and valued. They understand that relationships require discretion and careful pacing, and they do not take inappropriate liberties too early. They are better able to perceive and accurately interpret verbal and nonverbal feedback. In the event of conflict, they are able to call into play a number of adaptive social strategies such as humor, distraction, and negotiation to resolve conflicts. Popular children are skilled in modulating their language according to their audience. Moreover, they know how to market themselves: as competent cultural anthropologists, they understand the behaviors and appearances that are admired by their peers!

What can we say, then, about middle childhood development among children with spina bifida? Of course, no "typical" child exists, and different children are going to have different sets of attributes and vulnerabilities. Even though children with spina bifida vary as much as other children do, certain characteristics of cognitive development are shared by many affected children. These characteristics predispose children to certain learning disabilities and academic difficulties. Equally important are the social difficulties that many children with spina bifida encounter because of social isolation, lack of social skills, or a combination of these.

Learning Abilities and Disabilities

The diagnosis, assessment, and management of learning disabilities is a field so full of controversial issues that it is extremely difficult to address in sufficient depth. A good starting point is a definition: learning disabilities (note the plural) are a heterogeneous group of disorders of presumed neurologic origin that selectively interferes with the acquisition and use of listening, reading, speaking, writing, mathematics, and social skills.

The key concept here is that children, when we examine their language, memory, attention, visual-perceptual ability, and so forth, have a profile of strengths and weaknesses. As many as 10 to 20 percent of children have striking weaknesses or dysfunctions in one or more areas that are important for academic performance. If these selective areas of dysfunction are leading to significant academic underachievement, than we consider these children to have learning disabilities. For example, if a child has receptive language dysfunction that results in a considerable delay in reading comprehension and ability to follow instructions, then we would consider the child to have a language-based learning disability.

Of course, not every child with low achievement has a learning disability. The question is, How uneven is the profile, and how selective is the dysfunction? If a child has low achievement in all areas and shows dysfunction in most cognitive areas that are assessed, her or his overall cognitive ability or intellect is likely to be low—that is, the child may be a slow learner.

The definition of learning disabilities is one thing, but the diagnosis and assessment of learning disabilities is quite another! How do we determine whether a child's low academic achievement is due to a specific learning disability or due to overall low ability, depression, or some other cause? Historically, these thorny issues have been dealt with using a discrepancy formula, whereby some arbitrary discrepancy was set between IQ score (as a measure of overall ability) and achievement score, usually fifteen points. A child with an IQ of 100 and a reading standard score of 85 would be considered learning disabled (LD), whereas another child with an IQ of 95 and a reading score of 81 would not. Such rigid use of discrepancy criteria is problematic for a number of reasons. First, the fifteen-point cutoff is very arbitrary, and there is no justification in concluding that the former student has a problem that needs assisting, whereas the latter does not, or that the former student will respond to remedial educational approaches better than will the latter. Second, many students have specific dysfunctions that affect their performance on IQ tests to some extent, thereby depressing their scores and disqualifying them for assistance. In this way, many students with learning disabilities fall through the cracks of our educational system, failing to receive the assistance and intensive remediation efforts that they need for success. Furthermore, instead of trying to figure out the individual student's strengths and weaknesses and to determine his or her individual needs, regardless of labels, too much effort is wasted on deciding whether a student is to be labeled LD. Such an approach is overly simplistic and ultimately robs many struggling children of the opportunity to benefit from individualized educational approaches.

As the reader can tell, I have a bias in this field and strongly favor a nonlabeling approach that recognizes and celebrates diversity among children. This diversity is self-evident to those of us who are clinicians working with children. I think that assessment of children should be more than a sterile and routine effort to establish whether a fifteen-point discrepancy exists. Instead, it should provide a rich description of strengths and weaknesses across a range of functions, giving the classroom teachers useful information regarding the student's cognitive style, underutilized strengths, and classroom strategies that may be helpful to that student. I have been sensitized to these issues because I have occasionally had to battle to get a child assessed and appropriately served. An example of the kind of letter that I frequently write to the schools on behalf of struggling school-age children is shown in Figure 8.2. I shall return to issues of public law in education, due process, and special education in Chapter 11.

Common Learning Characteristics

As shown in Figure 2.9, children with spina bifida as a whole score about ten or fifteen points lower on IQ tests than a normal population of children. In other words, the mean (average) IQ is in the low average range (around 85–90), instead of hovering around 100. This is not to say that all such children will be in this range, and considerable spread exists in the range of IQs that I see in the patients in my clinic. I have several youngsters with IQ scores in the above average or superior range. Similarly, a significant proportion of children will test out in the mild range of mental retardation.

For most children with spina bifida, the Verbal IQ tends to be higher than the Performance IQ. In fact, a significant difference in this direction occurs twice as often in those with spina bifida as occurs in the normal population. Although some studies show that higher-level lesions are associated with lower scores, this association has too many exceptions to be very useful. Perhaps of more interest is the association of IQ scores with shunt complications. In McLone's study, children who did not have significant hydrocephalus and were not shunted had a mean IQ of 102 (McLone et al. 1982). Those who were shunted but had no shunt complications were not significantly different on testing (a mean IQ of 95). By contrast, those children who had shunt complications had a mean IQ of only 73. It would appear from this study that the mere presence of hydrocephalus is not in itself a major risk factor for intellectual development, but ventriculitis and other major shunt complications may lead to acquired brain injury and limit subsequent development.

Perhaps the most common learning trait among children with spina bifida could be characterized as a visual-perceptual learning disability. Such children tend to struggle most in math, in which spatial concepts and logical-mathematical and quantitative reasoning are elusive. They may have trouble in tasks involving design and construction, because they cannot easily visualize how something is going to look. Spatial planning prob-

Re: John Murphy
Date of birth: 9/28/82

Dear Ms. Brown,

John Murphy is a child with spina bifida in your school whom we follow for comprehensive health care in our clinic. Our team is multidisciplinary in nature, and I work closely with a psychologist regarding issues of learning and school problems. Our assessment of John leads us to suspect strongly that he has a learning disability.

Before giving you some specifics about John, I want to provide you background information regarding learning characteristics among children with spina bifida. Experts generally agree that children with spina bifida tend to have deficits in perceptual-motor development, such that the majority have discrepancies between higher Verbal IQ and lower Performance IQ scores. In our experience, children with spina bifida benefit greatly from special education interventions, both in the regular classrooms and in other settings. It is especially important that schools understand and address the specific learning problems of these children rather than erroneously attributing their problems to overall low ability. When applying a discrepancy formula for determining eligibility for LD services, it is usually more appropriate to use their Verbal IQ as a measure of cognitive ability rather than their Full Scale IQ, which is typically much lower because of the perceptual-motor difficulties.

Previous evaluation of John showed that he has visual-perceptual problems and slow processing speed. WISC-III Verbal IQ was 92, Performance IQ 82, and his standard score on the VMI was 80. By contrast, he had a score of 96 on the Peabody Picture Vocabulary Test. This profile is very consistent with the typical specific learning disability of spina bifida. We would therefore strongly urge you to proceed with educational testing as soon as possible, in order to provide more special education assistance for this child. If he does not meet discrepancy criteria, I would recommend provision of needed services under the Other Health Impairment category, because his neurologic condition is likely to interfere with his alertness, organization, and learning.

Yours sincerely,
Adrian Sandler, M.D.

Figure 8.2. A sample of a letter that may be helpful in obtaining appropriate special education services for a child with spina bifida

lems may also be evident in drawings and in samples of writing, in which children struggle with lines, margins, and organization on the page. Children with these problems can sometimes develop compensatory skills, often overrelying on rote memorization of math facts and procedures. Unfortunately, these strategies break down when children encounter fractions or other aspects of the math curriculum that require a firm grasp of the concepts.

Another common characteristic is that of the child with writing problems (dysgraphia). Although reading may be relatively strong, written output is slow, laborious, poorly organized, and often illegible. This kind of learning disability is often seen in children with fine-motor dysfunction and weaknesses in visual–fine-motor integration. Even if the child has excellent ideas to communicate, the strain of remembering and executing the letter formations, organizing the words into grammatical sentences, and developing a narrative sequence can lead to fatigue, loss of motivation, and decreasing academic self-esteem.

A third characteristic pattern of learning disability seen in some children with spina bifida is one that affects social performance rather than any specific area of academic performance. These children have subtle deficits in many areas of higher-order cognition. Their reasoning abilities, planning, judgment, strategy use, and cognitive flexibility are areas of weakness. Although their early progress in reading decoding may be adequate, they begin to show evidence of subtle comprehension difficulties. It is hard for them to understand complexity or to draw inferences. Scores on IQ tests are usually lower than expected because these talkative children have lively and outgoing personalities that may mask their underlying processing problems. The language characteristics of such children have been described as the "cocktail party syndrome." Though not a true syndrome, the descriptive term is apt for this kind of learning disability. "Cocktail party" speech is typically fluent but often irrelevant, perseverative, and full of social phrases and clichés. Many of these children assume an overfamiliarity, coming on strong and failing to take the perspective of the listener. Peers are apt to notice such lack of social skills and regard these children as weird or otherwise different.

These descriptions of characteristic profiles are prototypes, and many children may have elements of these but do not fit neatly into one category or another. Many others, of course, will be essentially average kids who are performing well both academically and socially. For those who are struggling in these domains, however, I have included a number of education management strategies in Chapter 11.

Attention Deficit Disorder

Attention deficit disorder is the most common kind of learning difficulty, affecting around 5 percent of all schoolchildren. The prevalence among children with spina bifida is not known with certainty, but I suspect it occurs somewhat more often than in the general population. Attention deficits are being recognized, diagnosed, and treated at increasing rates in the United States and elsewhere, but these troublesome symptoms have probably occurred for centuries. John Locke, in his book *On the Conduct of the Understanding* (1762), discussed the problems of "this wandering of the thoughts." In more recent times, many terms such as minimal brain dysfunction, hyperactivity, and attention-deficit hyperactivity disorder (ADHD) have been used to describe this common and perplexing problem (Figure 8.3).

A distinguishing feature of the condition is a tendency to be distracted easily. Many children may focus intently on their favorite television program or video game. When the subject matter is less exciting and alluring, however, their thoughts may wander uncontrollably, or they may be distracted by sights and sounds in the classroom or outside the window.

Some children with attention deficits are tremendously energetic and overactive. But many others have normal activity levels and are not unusually fidgety. Most of the children with spina bifida and attention deficits fall into this nonhyperactive group. One of the hallmarks of the condition is performance inconsistency: children might complete a math assignment correctly on Thursday but barely be able to start one on Friday. Grades and test scores are highly erratic and unpredictable. Because children do well once in a while, their parents and teachers assume that they should always work at that standard, and their failure to do so is often attributed to laziness or lack of motivation. A cycle of failure and frustration commonly ensues.

Another important characteristic of children with attention deficits is their tendency to be impulsive. They frequently omit the planning stages in their schoolwork, their behavior, and the things they say, which gets them into trouble, both socially and academically. Many children have a hurried work style, and in their efforts to rush through their work, they make impulsive and careless errors.

Attention deficits may occur in conjunction with other learning disabilities, and it is important not to make the mistake of attributing a child's problems to her or his attention deficits while ignoring the underlying learning disability. For many children with spina bifida, problems

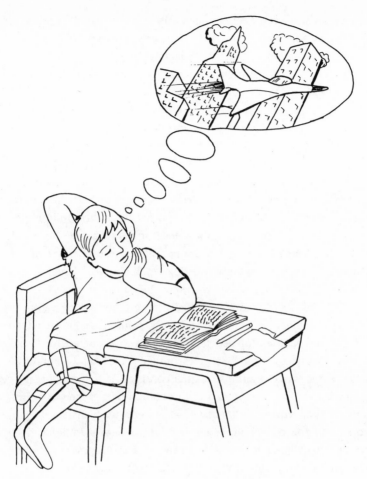

Figure 8.3. Attention deficit disorder (usually without hyperactivity) is a fairly common problem among children with spina
bifida.

with attention may be largely secondary to their visual-perceptual learning disability or simply reflect the fact that they do not understand what
is going on because they are in an inappropriate educational setting.

The diagnosis of attention deficit disorder rests heavily on an experienced clinician's careful history and exclusion of other important diag-
noses. It is especially important to consider whether other learning disabilities are present. Scales that rate the child's behavior in school and
other settings can be helpful, and the direct input from an observant
teacher can be invaluable. The use of computerized continuous perfor-

mance tests has become very popular. Although the validity of these tests has been called into question, I think that they can contribute to the assessment and diagnosis of attention deficits.

Most youngsters with attention deficits benefit from low doses of stimulant medication—Ritalin and Dexedrine are the most commonly prescribed, having been in use for over fifty years. Children do not become addicted to these drugs and experience few side effects if medication is used carefully and with appropriate supervision. Large numbers of children with spina bifida have been treated with Ritalin; generally, the results are favorable. In my experience, about a third show dramatic improvement in attention and classroom performance, often with enhancement of organizational skills and writing. Another third show mild improvements, and the remaining third show no improvement or develop troublesome side effects such as appetite suppression, headache, or irritability. Although stimulants can cause constipation, I have not found this to be a significant problem in children with spina bifida.

It is important to realize that medicines are not a panacea but only one part of a total management plan. Most children need to be helped to understand their attention deficits and to know that they are not "lazy" or "stupid." Parents too need help in learning how to foster their child's self-esteem while providing the structure, consistency, and support needed by their child. Education is the most important part of the management. Many children with attention deficits can be effectively managed by interventions in the classroom, sometimes without the additional help of medication, using such strategies as those given in Figure 11.2. To implement such strategies effectively, it is essential to develop an alliance between parents and schoolteachers.

Although children were once thought to outgrow their attention deficits, it is now recognized that at least half continue to have troublesome symptoms through adolescence and some even in adulthood. It is important to stress that the outcome for children with spina bifida and attention deficits is generally favorable. Many of these children have the potential to become successful and productive adults. It is vital that they are given the opportunity to succeed in school and avoid humiliation and demoralization. Given this support, the presence of attention deficits should not be a significant obstacle to future success.

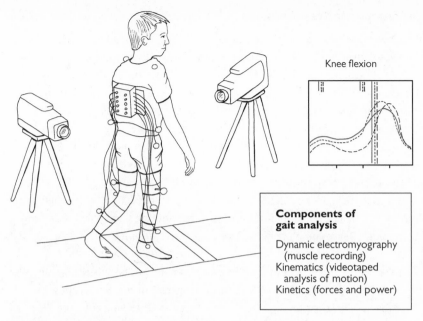

Knee flexion

Components of gait analysis

Dynamic electromyography
  (muscle recording)
Kinematics (videotaped
  analysis of motion)
Kinetics (forces and power)

Figure 8.4. Gait analysis: accurate analysis of the speed, forces, and movements of the lower limbs during walking can be very helpful in making decisions and planning treatment.

HABILITATION ISSUES

Gait Analysis

Gait analysis has had a major impact on medical decision making in the field of cerebral palsy. The idea of gait analysis is simple enough: Surface electrodes are placed on the skin over the key muscle groups used in walking, and activity in these groups is recorded and stored with the aid of a computer. In addition to recording muscle activity, a video camera is used to record joint motion, speed, and stride. Usually, markers are placed on the skin overlying key joints (ankle, knee, hip), so that as the person walks, the precise movements at the joints can be followed and analyzed (Figure 8.4). The intention of gait analysis is to provide objective data on which to base important therapeutic decisions. Many medical centers now use gait analysis in the management of children with spina bifida. The advocates of the technique have reported that they find it helpful in decisions about bracing, tendon transfers, and hip surgery. Technological advances, of course, do not substitute for experience and clinical skill in such decision making.

Physical Therapy and Adaptive PE

PE (physical education) is mandatory in schools for all students, including those with disabilities. Inclusion of children with spina bifida in PE programs presents a challenge to PE teachers, but most teachers clearly understand the importance of this challenge. First, a good workout keeps the child fit, leading to decreased obesity, stronger bones, and better bowel function. Second, a child develops a sense of teamwork through participation in group sports and games. Third, children develop the habit of recreation through regular participation in a variety of activities. I see many young adults with spina bifida and other disabilities who have good social skills and work skills but lack leisure skills, and it seems to me that their lives are a little poorer. Hopefully, an early introduction to physical activities through PE can help prevent a "couch potato" lifestyle!

There are countless adaptations that can be made to include children with disabilities in PE. Certain pieces of equipment can be substituted or the rules modified slightly to accommodate special needs. Sometimes, it is appropriate for the playing area to be reduced. As a general rule, the PE teacher should keep the spirit and overall purpose of the game the same. The use of wheelchairs, sports chairs, fun go-carts, and adapted bicycles should allow participation in most ball sports. Aerobics and other exercises involving dance and rhythm can be great fun. Swimming, bowling, and archery should all be accessible options. Orienteering, floor exercises, and exercise "circuits" can be challenging and may help the child with spina bifida develop spatial problem-solving skills. Leisure skills and recreational opportunities will be discussed in Chapter 11.

Certain precautions have to be taken to ensure safety. For example, the child with spina bifida who has no foot sensation needs protective footwear (socks or diving booties). I think that children with shunts need to be carefully supervised when doing tumbling and gymnastics to avoid traumatizing the shunt. The schools should have a teacher of adaptive PE who can provide special consultation to PE teachers regarding ideas for adaptations and the need for special precautions.

There should also be communication between the child's physical therapist and the teachers responsible for PE. The physical therapy (PT) needs of the child can be met to some extent during PE: instead of using PT exercises, certain sensorimotor activities can be incorporated into PE classes. Indeed, creative physical therapists have worked with classroom teachers to integrate therapy into music, drama, math, and science!

A Word about Independence and Continence

A few years ago, I was involved in a research study of social competence in elementary school–age children with spina bifida. We were interested in finding out what factors were important in predicting how well children did socially. One of the strong associations that we found was between social competence and continence: the children who were reliably dry and out of diapers were doing better socially. This result was not very surprising. After all, it is socially humiliating to have "accidents" or to have an odor of urine. For a child who is five or younger, these things hardly matter, and although getting out of diapers is a source of pride, still wearing them evokes little more than a shrug from peers. Not so in first grade, where the social stakes are high. For these reasons, the establishment of continence becomes a critical habilitation goal for the child in the early school years.

Clean Intermittent Catheterization

About 95 percent of children with myelomeningocele have a neurogenic bladder. They are unable to perceive bladder fullness and lack the neurologic integrity to have coordinated contraction of the bladder muscle and opening of the bladder sphincter. Most have uninhibited bladder contractions, which may be accompanied by high bladder pressures. Some may be able to empty partially by straining, but the emptying is incomplete. This predisposes them to urinary tract infections (UTIs). The combination of high bladder pressures and infection may place the kidneys at risk. Indeed, about twenty years ago many children with spina bifida died from renal failure.

In 1971, Dr. Lapides and his colleagues revolutionized the management of spina bifida. Like so many great medical advances, his was a simple idea. By passing a catheter several times a day, he reasoned, it should be possible to get complete emptying and thereby protect the kidneys. It proved to be highly effective and also provided an additional benefit: many were able to achieve continence.

Clean intermittent catheterization (CIC) should be done five to six times a day, which works out to be every three or four waking hours. Although this may seem very frequent, most of us are accustomed to urinating at least as often as this. A typical schedule for catheterization in the school-age child is as follows: 7:00 A.M., 10:00 A.M., 2:00 P.M., 6:00 P.M., and 9:30 P.M. The procedure should take only five minutes or less, and like everything else, the more often you do the catheterization, the faster you

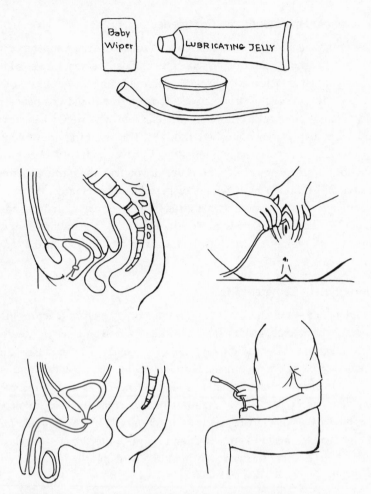

Figure 8.5. Essentials of clean intermittent catheterization

get! At the spina bifida camp, we've had about twenty-five kids lining up outside the "Med Shed," needing to be cathed before breakfast. It's amazing how efficient one can get with experience!

Figure 8.5 shows the catheterization procedure in males and females. For many parents, doing it the first few times can be very intimidating, but with good instruction and supervision, the feelings of insecurity soon pass. First, make sure you have the necessary equipment: a suitable catheter, a box of wipes, K-Y Jelly, a mild liquid soap, and a container for the urine. Hands should be washed, but gloves and sterile technique are not necessary.

It doesn't really matter what the catheter is made of, but most use catheters made of plastic. Some women use small metal catheters. Red "rubber" catheters are not usually made of latex, but some are and should not be used by children with spina bifida. Make sure that the catheter is of sufficient size. Most children can pass a 10 or 12 French gauge catheter. All too often, I have seen children using size 8 or smaller and thus having to wait for several minutes for the bladder to empty, or more common, they remove the catheter before the bladder is empty and then get infections.

CIC Procedure

Begin by wiping the genitals clean. For the male, hold the penis in one hand, wipe the urethral opening and then the rest of the head of the penis. For the uncircumsized male, it is better to pull back the foreskin (for very young boys whose foreskins do not retract fully, just do so partially so the catheter can be introduced into the urethra). For females, hold the labia apart with one hand to expose the urethra. Look carefully to identify the urethra. Then wipe from the direction of the clitoris down toward the anus. For both sexes, repeat the cleaning a total of three times, using a different part of the cloth with each wipe.

Next, introduce the catheter gently into the urethra. For males, use a little K-Y Jelly on the tip of the catheter for lubrication; for females, this is optional. One question that arises commonly (and can usually be discerned from the pained expression on a father's face!) is, "Will it hurt?" Almost always, the answer is no, although some youngsters put up a struggle the first time. Very rarely, individuals with preserved sensation may find the procedure uncomfortable; thus the use of a little lidocaine gel as lubricant may be helpful. The catheter should be advanced gently into the urethra until urine begins to flow (not drip) from the catheter: for boys, this may be about four to seven inches, and for girls, about one to three inches. There may be some resistance to passage of the catheter just before entering the bladder if the sphincter muscles are tight, which can usually be easily overcome with steady pressure. Another commonly asked question is, "Can it do any harm?" Again, if done gently, CIC is remarkably safe and free of complications. Moreover, most children can be harmed by *not* catheterizing. A few specks of blood may occasionally be seen in the urine from a slight scratch of the urethra, but this scratch heals easily without treatment. Rarely, I have seen the development of a "false passage," which is a blind-ending outpouching of the urethra, into which the catheter tends to slip, with resultant difficulty in catheterization. This rare complication needs the attention of a urologist.

Urine will start to flow when the catheter is in the bladder. If urine does not flow, it is because the catheter is not in the bladder. (In boys, no flow usually means the catheter has not passed through the sphincter; in girls, the catheter may have slipped into the vagina.) Let urine flow under gravity into a collecting container. Remember that urine will not flow up-hill, so make sure that the container is as low as possible. In this way, the bladder will be completely emptied. Usually, bladder capacities are in the range of 200 to 300 cc. A container with volumes marked on it can be helpful in assessing the success of the catheterization. Once the flow has stopped, it is a good idea to have the child sit up, which can help drain any additional urine.

Remove the catheter gently, washing it with warm, soapy water as the hands are washed. Rinse the catheter inside and out with running water; shake the excess water from inside the catheter and then dry the outside with a clean paper towel. Catheters need not be sterilized, although some like to boil the catheters for ten minutes or place them in water to which antiseptic chemicals have been added. The catheter can then be stored in a clean and dry container, such as a jar, plastic ziplock bag, toothbrush holder, or so on, until the next use.

Pharmacological Management of Incontinence

The majority of children with spina bifida have an unstable bladder muscle which has uninhibited contractions (spasms) and which fails to relax to allow adequate filling. To relax the bladder and make it more compli-ant, medication is usually necessary. These medicines (called anticholin-ergics) include oxybutynin (Ditropan), propantheline (Probanthine), and imipramine (Tofranil). Figure 8.6 shows the actions of medicines com-monly used in the management of the neurogenic bladder.

Before they enter school, we put children on a program of CIC so that they will be dry. If their bladders are noncompliant, they will prob-ably fail to achieve continence on CIC alone, having leaking of urine be-tween catheterizations. Starting them on an anticholinergic medication may allow sufficient bladder relaxation to enable them to go three to four hours without leaking. Some children have satisfactory bladder compli-ance on just one of these medicines, whereas others may need more than one medicine. The drug used most commonly is Ditropan, which is avail-able in tablet or liquid form. Like all anticholinergics, it can cause several side effects, including dry mouth, flushing, heat intolerance, constipa-tion, and drowsiness. However, most children are able to tolerate a dose of 2.5–5 mg three times a day without developing troublesome side effects. For those who do have severe flushing or dry mouth, it may be possible to

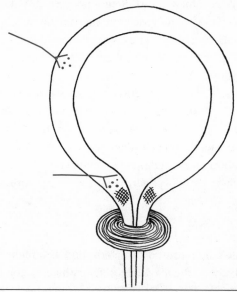

Medication	Mechanism	Usual dosage	Side effects
Oxybutynin (Ditropan)	Anticholinergic —relaxes bladder muscle	2.5–5 mg 2–4 times/day	Flushing Heat intolerance Dry mouth
Propantheline (Probanthine)	Anticholinergic —relaxes bladder muscle	7.5–15 mg 2–3 times/day	Same as above
Phenylpropanolamine (Ornade)	Alpha-adrenergic —tightens internal sphincter	75 mg 1–2 times/day	Sedation, confusion Rapid heart rate
Pseudoephedrine (Sudafed)	Alpha-adrenergic —tightens internal sphincter	15–30 mg 2–3 times/day	Same as above
Imipramine (Tofranil)	Antidepressant with anticholinergic effects on bladder	10–25 mg 1–2 times/day	Danger in overdose Dry mouth, dizziness, blurred vision, constipation

Figure 8.6. Pharmacological management of the neurogenic bladder

avoid these side effects by crushing a quarter or a half tablet of Ditropan, dissolving it in 5 cc of water, and then instilling this directly into the bladder through the catheter after the bladder has been drained. Studies have shown that this treatment is moderately effective and reduces side effects. Unfortunately, it may be inconvenient, adding yet one more step to day-to-day management.

Although imipramine has a direct effect on the bladder muscle, this drug is better known for a quite different purpose: it is an antidepressant medication that is sometimes used to treat depression, anxiety, and even attention deficits in children. The doses that are used for these purposes are typically two or three times higher than the doses used to treat the neurogenic bladder.

Some children have wetting between catheterizations because the bladder neck is wide open and the sphincter alone cannot hold back the urine. Such children will tend to leak urine, even when the bladder pressures are not high. Sometimes the open bladder neck can be treated with a different class of medication that stimulates the sphincter muscles to tighten. These medicines include pseudoephedrine (Sudafed), ephedrine, and phenylpropanolamine (Ornade).

How Dry Is "Dry"?

Although some children need catheterization as a medical necessity to protect their kidneys, the main reason for catheterization is the achievement of continence. The objective of beginning catheterization and anticholinergic medication around school entry is to be dry. What proportion of children with spina bifida will achieve urinary continence? This question is not as easy to answer as it seems. The problem is that people have different standards, and what is sufficiently dry to one may be unacceptable to another. Furthermore, I know that some families I see in clinic don't want to disappoint me and others on the team, and when I ask, "Is she dry in between caths?" I may get a positive response because they know that's the answer I want to hear! I would like to see all our schoolchildren be reliably dry and out of diapers, but I know that this goal is unreasonable. In reality, around 50–90 percent of children will be reliably dry or will have only occasional episodes of wetting. It is hard to know for sure, because some may say they're dry and just use pads or diapers for security, when in fact they are damp all day.

Incontinence is one of those things that is uncomfortable to talk about. It's hard for doctors to admit treatment failures; it's difficult for parents to confront this stigmatizing aspect of the disability; and it's hard for children to admit they're different. Thus the problem is ignored, and the child and family just accept things the way they are. If occasional or infrequent incontinence is acceptable to the child and family, then the clinician should go along with it. If this wetness means a feeling of helplessness, hopelessness, and resignation to a state of complete incontinence, then it is up to the clinician to explore further. It is important that physicians and nurses establish a relationship with their patients and an environment in

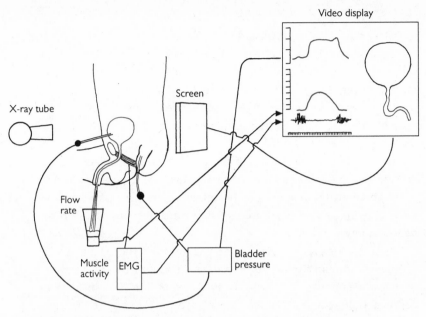

Figure 8.7. Urodynamic studies may include the measurement of bladder pressure, volume, and muscle activity (EMG).

which it is comfortable to talk about these crucial issues. Parents and children need to be encouraged to bring up concerns about continence in clinic. Almost always there is something than can be done to improve the situation.

When a child fails to achieve an acceptable degree of continence on a bladder program of catheterization and anticholinergic medication, there may be several explanations. The family may not be following through with the catheterizations, or they may be doing them inconsistently or too infrequently. Children who are on self-catheterization may *say* they're doing it but in reality are skipping caths. Many children may not be emptying the bladder, perhaps because they are using a small catheter or withdrawing the catheter too soon. Such problems can be remedied easily by carefully reviewing and checking techniques in the clinic.

Not infrequently, persistent incontinence may be due to problems that are not so easily remedied. Perhaps a child's bladder is of very small capacity and unable to hold more than 150–200 cc. Such children may need additional anticholinergic therapy or even require surgery. Urodynamic studies can be of great help in sorting out these problems and allowing rational management (Figure 8.7).

Surgical Management of Incontinence

If bladder capacity is too small and the bladder is too noncompliant, even on maximal anticholinergic therapy, continence may be achieved with surgery to enlarge the bladder (augmentation). The most common augmentation procedure is the enterocystoplasty, in which the bladder is opened up and a part of the large intestine, the cecum, is sutured to the open bladder, dramatically increasing its capacity. The large augmented bladder then functions as a floppy reservoir, which must be emptied by catheterization. One variation of this operation is the Mitrofanoff procedure, in which the appendix is used to connect the augmented bladder to the abdominal wall at or near the umbilicus, such that the bladder is catheterized through a small stoma. This is sometimes known as a continence ostomy.

Augmentation procedures can be very successful in the treatment of incontinence and can also help protect the kidneys if there is severe reflux. As in any major operation, there is a small risk of rupture or breakdown. Fortunately, long-term results have been good, and serious complications are uncommon. There appears to be a high incidence of stone formation in augmented bladders, possibly related to the excessive mucus produced by the segment of intestine.

Another possible cause of persistent incontinence is that the bladder neck is wide open, allowing leakage even at low pressures. Attempts to manage this with medications may be unsuccessful, and there are numerous surgical operations designed to elevate or tighten the bladder neck or to implant an artificial sphincter.

Teaching Self-Catheterization

There is no specific age at which a child is ready to learn self-catheterization. If CIC begins at five years of age, most six-year-old children should be participating to some extent. Some children may pick up the skills quickly and easily and have the ability to self-catheterize by the age of six or seven. For anatomical reasons, it is easier for boys to find the urethra than it is for girls. The use of a mirror and a good light may be helpful in showing a girl her anatomy, but most manage well if they are taught a "touch technique," using their fingertips to locate the clitoris and then move down until they find the opening of the urethra.

Positioning is an important consideration. Braces can be modified to allow abduction of the hip to permit a girl to catheterize. If the hips are tight and difficult to abduct, it may be helpful to abduct them manu-

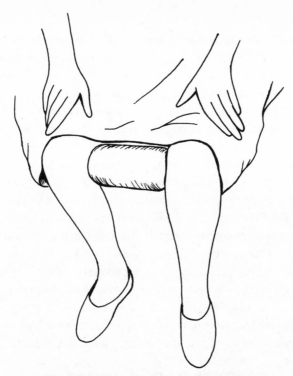

Figure 8.8. Self-catheterization: using a canister of
baby wipes to hold legs apart

ally and then place an object like a baby wipe canister between the knees
to keep them abducted (see Figure 8.8). Self-catheterization may be done
while sitting on the toilet or in the wheelchair. For other boys and girls, it
may be easier to do the job while standing up and leaning their knees up
against the toilet for balance.

Problems with hand control, eye-hand coordination, attention, and
sequencing can all interfere with the acquisition of these skills. Practice
and supervision, along with the use of prompting and cues, should allow
the child to make progress, despite these dysfunctions. Even if the child
lacks the skills to be independent in self-catheterization, he or she can still
be responsible for gathering the supplies, assisting with cleaning, removing the catheter, and helping with diapering and/or dressing. These early
steps toward independence should be rewarding and contribute greatly to
a sense of self-esteem.

Bladder Stimulation

More recently there have been some new developments in the management of the neurogenic bladder that are based on the techniques of biofeedback. The central idea is that children who have some physical sensations from the bladder can learn what it feels like to have bladder fullness and, over time, can learn techniques to initiate contractions and thereby empty their bladders. Such bladder stimulation programs will not work for everyone but have potential for those children with some bladder sensation. The program requires an intelligent child with a very committed family. The process takes at least one month of daily biofeedback in order to develop adequate sensation of bladder fullness. The data indicate that just over half the children who were candidates for bladder stimulation developed adequate sensation, and only a very small proportion, if any, developed urinary control (Dector, Snyder, and Rosvanis 1992; Boone, Roehrborn, and Hurt 1992). In our clinic, several children with spina bifida have spontaneously developed control of bladder emptying without rigorous biofeedback, and so I wonder if at least some of those who succeeded with the bladder stimulation programs might not have developed bladder control anyway. Clearly, this matter needs further study.

Management of the Neurogenic Bowel

Most children with spina bifida retain stool and develop constipation. Lack of mobility, reduced dietary fiber, and decreased motility of the bowel contribute to this problem. As a result, stool can build up in the rectum and colon, yet most children lack the sensation of rectal fullness. Constipation can cause some medical problems, including a tendency to develop urinary tract infections. The importance of constipation as far as habilitation is concerned, however, is that it can greatly interfere with the development of bowel continence. There are many different methods for children with spina bifida to establish bowel control, but they can all be thwarted by constipation. It is therefore essential to treat constipation when it occurs and to try to prevent it from reoccurring.

In the three- to five-year-old child, it may be possible to establish satisfactory bowel control through a combination of dietary measures to prevent constipation and teaching the young child to strain on the potty chair after meals. Although sometimes very successful, such a program requires adult supervision and in no way guarantees that the bowel movements are going to occur at the right times. When a child enters school, it is usually preferable to have her or him on a bowel program that gives

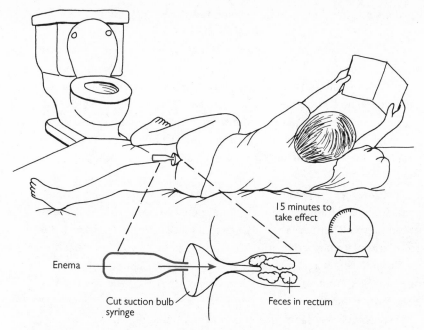

Enema

Cut suction bulb
syringe

15 minutes to
take effect

Feces in rectum

Figure 8.9. Regular administration of an enema may be an important part of a bowel program.

more reliable and complete emptying of the rectum at home, so the child can be secure about not having "accidents" at school. Because it is an enormous social disadvantage to be in diapers or to have incontinence of stool at school, a bowel program that works is important.

In our clinic, we usually teach parents to use bisacodyl, a laxative that triggers the rectum to empty completely. A one-ounce bisacodyl enema is used most commonly, although it may also be given in suppository form (Dulcolax). If the anal sphincter is weak, the enema tends to run straight out unless the buttocks are held closed. An adaptation is to administer the enema through a suction bulb that has been cut in half (see Figure 8.9). If the suppository is used, it should be taken out of the refrigerator long enough to warm to room temperature. The suppository should be inserted high in the rectum and held up against the bowel wall for a few seconds before removing the finger. The enema or suppository can be inserted with the child lying on one side, with the knee bent; the child should be encouraged to stay lying down in that position for about fifteen to twenty minutes while the bisacodyl is taking effect. Then the child should transfer to the toilet (or potty chair) and strain to empty the rectum. Evacuation times are variable, but most can get good emptying in about fifteen minutes. The child should learn to be responsible for wiping and the like.

When starting on such a program, it may be necessary to follow this procedure every night for a week or two. But once the program is established, it is usually possible to empty the rectum sufficiently so as to go without a bowel movement for at least two days. In other words, the enema would be repeated two nights later, by which time the rectum would have filled again with stool. Most children on such a program are essentially free of "accidents" if they have enemas every other night or about three times a week.

There are many other bowel regimens that work well for different children. Some children are able to maintain continence by timed Valsalva (straining) after dinner. Some use glycerin suppositories instead of the bowel stimulant bisacodyl. Still others use the enema continence catheter, through which a saline enema of about 20 cc/kg (about half a liter) is run into the rectum. This system uses a balloon to retain the saline in the bowel until emptying.

There are many reasons why efforts to get a child on a bowel program might be frustrating and difficult. Compliance is a major issue and one that I will address in the next chapter. The two most common reasons for stool incontinence in a child who is on a bowel program are the return of constipation and dietary indiscretion. It is essential to examine the abdomen for evidence of stool and if necessary to get an X-ray of the abdomen. If the colon is loaded with stool, then the soft stool above this area may pass from the rectum unpredictably and with embarrassing consequences. Certain foods are very likely to stimulate the bowel and lead to incontinence. The main culprits include chocolate, pizza, tomatoes, corn, Kool-Aid, and candy. An astute parent knows precisely what triggers bowel movements in his or her child and keeps reminding the child to avoid these foods.

There is no perfect bowel program, but the adherence to a program definitely improves the chances of reliable bowel continence. It is important to find a system that achieves good results and is acceptable, working with the clinic team to find solutions to problems that may arise along the way.

Medical Issues

Growth and Growth Problems

Short stature is common in children with spina bifida and is probably caused by many factors (Greene et al. 1985). Eighty percent of those with lesions at

L3 or higher have short stature (recumbent length at less than the third percentile), compared with only about 40 percent of those with lower lesions. Undoubtedly, small lower limbs, spinal deformities, and scoliosis contribute to short stature. Scoliosis makes measurement of growth velocity difficult in these children, and many advocate arm span as the best measurement of their linear growth. Many older children have early and rapidly progressing puberty, which leads to advancement of bone age and further limitation of growth potential.

Differences in frequency and amplitude of growth hormone secretion have been reported in seven children with myelomeningocele (Rotenstein, Reigel, and Flom 1989). These children were treated with growth hormone in an uncontrolled study. Growth rates increased from 1.7 cm/year to 7.9 cm/year in six of the children after six months of growth hormone therapy. One child's therapy was discontinued because of progression of her scoliosis. Another subject developed hypothyroidism after three months of therapy.

The essential questions regarding the impact of growth hormone therapy have not been addressed in research studies. It is not unexpected to see augmentation of growth with short-term treatment, but is there a meaningful change in predicted adult height? Moreover, those children who are most likely to be significantly growth retarded are children with high-lumbar or thoracic lesions. These children are usually in wheelchairs, and one has to wonder whether moderate increases in sitting height are likely to have a major impact on the perceptions of peers and the social or physical self-esteem of the children. For ambulatory children who are acutely aware of their small stature, growth hormone therapy may well have a role. Children who are considered to be candidates for growth hormone therapy should be closely monitored for the development of hypothyroidism. Significant scoliosis is a contraindication to therapy, as this may substantially increase as a result of growth hormone affecting the growth of abnormal and asymmetric vertebrae. There is also a theoretical risk of symptomatic tethering of the spine during a period of rapid growth.

Until further evidence is available, growth hormone therapy should not be used indiscriminately in children with spina bifida and short stature. Longitudinal data on larger numbers of children are needed before the safety of such therapy in this population is established.

Precocious Puberty

We are all familiar with the dramatic changes and hormonal surges that occur with puberty and the striking variation in puberty development

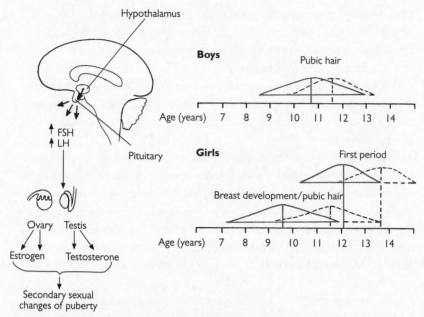

Figure 8.10. Hormonal control of puberty. Early puberty in boys and girls with spina bifida is shown by the curves. The peak of the curves represents the average age at which particular stages of puberty occur in children with spina bifida (red) and children without spina bifida (black). Boys with spina bifida reach puberty about one year earlier than boys without the condition; the difference for girls is about two years.

that is evident among children at ages ten through fourteen years. One visit to a sixth grade classroom provides dramatic evidence of the effects of sex hormones! Puberty is ushered in by a complex sequence of neuroendocrine adjustments in the brain. The hypothalamus and pituitary gland experience major changes, and circulating levels of sex hormones increase dramatically. These hormones in turn act on the sex organs, which undergo the obvious and familiar changes of puberty development, stimulating the growth spurt that occurs during these years (Figure 8.10). The process of puberty occurs a little earlier in girls than in boys. Breast development begins at a mean age of 11.5 years, and menarche (the first menstrual period) begins around 13.5 years. The growth spurt of puberty occurs at about 12 years in girls and 13 years in boys.

In children with spina bifida (and similarly in children with hydrocephalus for other reasons) there is frequently a premature activation of the hypothalamus and pituitary, and thus puberty begins early. Precocious puberty is defined as the onset of puberty before eight years of age in girls and before the age of nine in boys. In one study, seven of fifty-two (13 percent) girls with spina bifida had precocious puberty.

There are two main concerns about going into puberty early. The first is a medical one: in addition to premature sexual development, there is premature bone development, which causes the growth plates of the bones to mature and fuse early, thereby limiting further growth. The second concern is a psychological one, in that some children may not be ready for these changes. Breast development, acne, and the onset of periods may exaggerate a girl's feelings of being different and further isolate her from her peer group. Gentle support and developmentally appropriate sex education and preparation for the changes that are underway may be sufficient to prevent major adjustment difficulties. Books and other educational resources are available to help prepare children for the changes of puberty (Sloan 1993).

Referral to an endocrinologist should be considered for children with precocious puberty, especially if the bone age is advancing rapidly and concerns exist about adult height. Medroxyprogesterone may be useful to slow the progression of puberty but does not have an effect on height. In recent years, synthetic analogues of Gn-RH (gonadotropin-releasing hormone) have been used successfully to suppress the hormonal changes of puberty, but there are no published studies involving children with spina bifida.

Nutrition and Prevention of Obesity

The motor paralysis of spina bifida leads to a decrease in the daily amount of calories that are burned. Because caloric needs are lower, there is a tendency to gain weight. We live in a "fast food" society, in which we face constant pressure to indulge in tasty foods that are inexpensive, attractive, easy to obtain, and bad news nutritionally! As children become more independent during the school years, the opportunities to indulge increase dramatically, and it becomes harder for parents to monitor and influence food choices. It is not surprising that at least 20 percent of six- to twelve-year-old children with spina bifida are obese.

In the clinic, we monitor children's height and weight very closely, plotting the measurements on growth charts. Of course, such charts can be misleading because of the short stature and other linear growth characteristics outlined above. Changes in the weight/height ratio over time can be especially helpful in determining whether a child is gaining too much weight. It may also be beneficial to measure skinfold thickness in a standardized way (Figure 8.11).

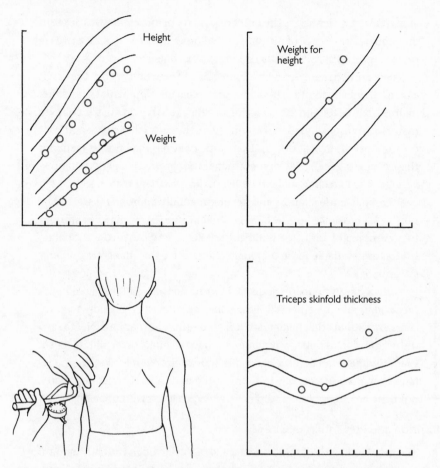

Figure 8.11. The development of obesity in a child with spina bifida. Recordings of height, weight, and skinfold thickness are charted over time on growth charts, providing reliable evidence of obesity.

The diagnosis of obesity is a lot easier than the treatment. Time and time again I see parents in the clinic who say, "I know what you're going to say, Dr. Sandler!" Just telling someone every six months to lose weight is not likely to do much good. Eating patterns and behaviors that contribute to the problem are often entrenched in the family, and others in the family may also be overweight. Success depends on the following ingredients: family commitment and involvement, parent and child nutrition education, aerobic exercise, and feedback and supervision.

First and foremost, to seek a solution, the family needs to accept that excess weight is a problem. If the parents are not committed to making some changes, forget it! I find it helpful to concentrate on the positive, emphasizing the benefits that await the whole family by adopting better nutritional and exercise habits, rather than focusing on the negative and trying to use scare tactics. If an overweight mother and her child can be encouraged to embark on a weight loss program together, this dramatically increases the likelihood of success.

Nutrition education is very important. We health care professionals often assume that everyone knows that fried chicken and potato chips are high in fat, but this is not always the case. Advertising can be misleading, and thousands of dieters choose a salad and then pour two hundred calories of salad dressing on top of it! Parents need to know that sweetened tea, sodas, candy, french fries, and fast food are out; that low-calorie, low-fat options and dietetic substitutes can be bought in the grocery store; and that delicious food can be prepared in new ways. As a general guideline, children with spina bifida should be on a diet of approximately 10 kCal per cm, or around 1,200 to 1,600 kCals per day.

Children also need nutrition education. One system that has been successfully used with children is the Stop-Caution-Go system, where common foods are listed in three groups. Green is for Go and includes those low-calorie foods that can be eaten with impunity. Orange is for Caution, for those foods that can be eaten in moderation—perhaps two such choices per day. Red is for Stop, which includes doughnuts and french fries—food choices that are to be avoided on all but very special occasions (and only then under supervision).

I feel like a broken record writing about the benefits of exercise, but the simple truth is that the combination of aerobic exercise and a weight-reducing diet is effective. Walking, pushing distances in the wheelchair on the track, aerobics, swimming, and rowing are all activities that I have seen children with spina bifida do successfully. Increasingly, there exist opportunities to participate in athletics and facilities that are accessible for disabled children. If nothing is readily available in the community, using a videotape for wheelchair aerobics can get your youngster moving.

As in other initiatives to change behavior, feedback is vitally important. Weight charts on the wall, showing the number of pounds lost week by week, can give visual reinforcement to a child and provide the encouragement to continue in his or her efforts.

Bacteriuria and Urinary Tract Infection

Urinary tract infections are common and a significant cause of illness in children with spina bifida. There is a spectrum of severity of infection in

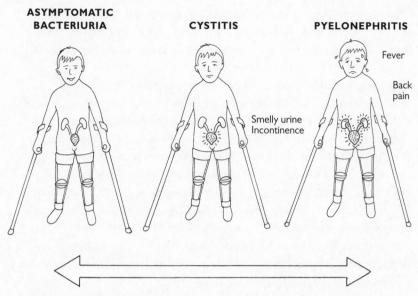

Figure 8.12. The spectrum of urinary tract infections. Bacteria in the bladder may be "normal" and completely harmless for some, whereas severe infection going up to the kidneys may require vigorous antibiotic therapy and hospitalization for others.

children with neurogenic bladders (Figure 8.12). Most commonly, there is asymptomatic infection of the bladder (asymptomatic bacteriuria): a child feels fine, but the urine in the bladder contains bacteria. If the bladder infection is acute, there may be some inflammation of the bladder (cystitis), accompanied by mild symptoms. For example, children with cystitis may have incontinence because their bladders are irritable and contract with low urine volumes. They may carry the odor of smelly urine, which has social consequences. If the bladder infection is severe, they may feel unwell, complain of abdominal or back pain, or develop a fever. Under some circumstances, the infection may ascend up the ureters and into the kidneys (pyelonephritis). Kidney infections are usually associated with high fever, vomiting, or other signs of serious infection and have the potential to damage the kidneys and leave permanent kidney scars.

Asymptomatic bacteriuria is to be expected in children with neurogenic bladders (Schlager and Dilks 1995). One of the most common mistakes that primary care doctors make is the overtreatment of asymptomatic bacteriuria in children with spina bifida. In a child who is feeling fine, who is not having an increase in wetting, and whose kidneys are not at risk, I do not recommend treatment with antibiotics just because there are bacteria in the urine. The use of antibiotics in this situation is likely to select out resistance to antibiotics in the bacterial population; thus the next culture will show a different strain of bacteria that is resistant to the antibiotics that were used. If the doctor responds by choosing another antibiotic, this too will select resistant organisms; eventually the child is likely to carry highly resistant bacteria in the bladder. If he or she should develop a symptomatic infection, few or no options may be left for oral therapy, and the infection may be considerably harder to treat.

Generally, it is important to screen the urine periodically for bacteriuria. In our clinic, about 30 to 40 percent of the children have asymptomatic bacteriuria when they come in. Those who are constipated are more likely to have evidence of bacteriuria. We use dipsticks to screen for nitrites and leukocyte esterase and culture only those who are positive on either or both of these tests. The positive predictive value of these dipstick screening tests is about .7, and the negative predictive value is about .9. Annual renal ultrasound examinations provide an excellent means of assessing the state of the upper tracts. If the kidneys and ureters remain normal, without evidence of hydronephrosis and with normal interim renal growth, this is very reassuring evidence of stability. If renal ultrasound suggests deterioration, in the sense of development or worsening of caliectasis or hydronephrosis, we would usually proceed with VCUG (video-cystourethrography) or a nuclear scan to look for evidence of reflux and/or renal scarring.

If a child with a neurogenic bladder and bacteriuria is completely asymptomatic and has no evidence of reflux, antibiotic therapy is generally not indicated. If there are symptoms, then the drugs most often used are trimethoprim-sulfa (Septra) or nitrofurantoin (Macrodantin), for seven days. Other oral antibiotics may be indicated according to the sensitivities of the bacteria isolated from the urine culture. Children with pyelonephritis generally require intravenous antibiotics for adequate treatment.

For the child with reflux, the situation is different because the bladder infection is much more likely to ascend up to the kidneys and cause damage. These children should be on prophylactic antibiotics (Septra or Macrodantin at night) to help prevent infections, and if they develop bacteriuria it should be appropriately treated with antibiotics.

Tethering, Detethering, and Retethering

In the course of normal childhood growth, the spinal cord ascends within the spinal canal. The end of the cord (the conus) is at the bottom of L3 at birth and is around the top of L2 by adolescence. In spina bifida and other congenital spinal cord conditions, the abnormal spinal cord tends to get stuck in a lower position and tethered to scar tissue or bony deformities. This leads to stretching of the cord and its blood vessels, which may produce damage to the cord, further interfering with nerve function. This pathological fixation of the spinal cord in an abnormal position may be associated with hydromyelia (fluid cyst in the cord), cord lipomas, or other spinal cord problems (Figure 8.13).

Tethering may occur in the preschooler but more commonly becomes clinically apparent in the six- to twelve-year-old child. Some of the clinical features are shown in Figure 8.13: progressive deterioration in gait; loss of strength, hamstring tightness, and orthopedic deformity (especially increasing valgus deformity of the foot); early development of rapidly increasing scoliosis; such postural changes as increasing lumbar lordosis; back and leg pain; change in urologic function (such as needing to catheterize more frequently, incontinence, increase in uninhibited contractions on urodynamics); and changes in bowel function, such as fecal soiling.

The diagnosis of tethering is essentially made on clinical grounds. In some cases, the symptoms come on quite suddenly and are fairly easy to recognize. Unfortunately, the symptoms can often arise insidiously, and by the time they are recognized, there is little one can do. One teenager in our clinic was born with L3-level spina bifida, and his parents were told he would walk. Between the ages of two and eight he had gradually increasing scoliosis and loss of function. Functionally, he now has a T5 paralysis because of severe and intractable tethering. Although the MRI scan of the spine is very good at accurately showing a low-lying conus, such a finding is necessary but not sufficient for a diagnosis of tethered cord. Because surgical treatment of tethered cord may have complications, it is important to obtain other supportive evidence that symptomatic tethering exists. Detailed manual muscle testing should be carried out on regular visits and the findings recorded to provide the documentation of change over time. Electrophysiologic testing using such tools as EMG (electromyography), SSEVP (somatosensory-evoked potentials), and urodynamics may provide additional evidence of acquired neurologic dysfunction.

The treatment of tethering should be undertaken only by an experienced pediatric neurosurgeon. In recent years, newer techniques including laser surgery and microdissection have been developed and used with good effect in these operations. When the tethering is accompanied by severe spasticity, some surgeons advocate doing selective rhizotomy in addition to detethering. The results of the surgery are generally quite favorable. Re-

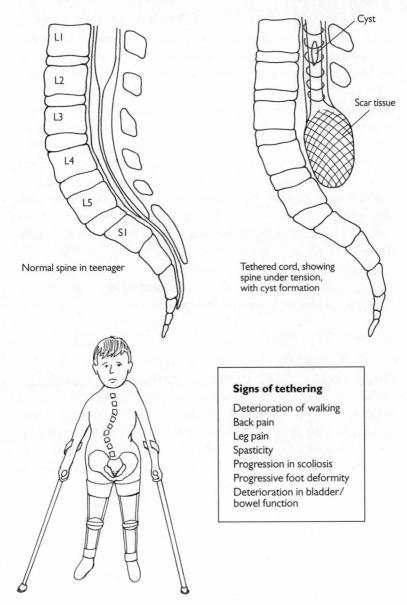

Normal spine in teenager

Cyst

Scar tissue

Tethered cord, showing spine under tension, with cyst formation

Signs of tethering

Deterioration of walking
Back pain
Leg pain
Spasticity
Progression in scoliosis
Progressive foot deformity
Deterioration in bladder/
bowel function

Figure 8.13. Tethering of the spinal cord may be associated with other spinal cord abnormalities.

lief of pain is a very likely outcome. For those with symptoms of fairly recent onset, there is a very good chance of improved muscle function and
decreased spasticity. There is some evidence that the procedure may also
improve bladder compliance (Gross et al. 1993). Improvement of scoliosis is
likely to occur in more than 50 percent of children with low-lumbar myelomeningocele and relatively mild curves. The prospects for improvement of
scoliosis in those with thoracic spina bifida are much less favorable, however, especially if the scoliosis is severe or there is associated hydromyelia.

Unfortunately, much of the published data regarding tethering are rather
weak. Although short-term results of surgery are good, few long-term
studies examine functional outcomes in those who have the procedure
compared with those who do not. In one series, around 20 percent of
those who had detethering surgery had recurrence of symptoms of sufficient severity that repeat detethering was undertaken. The best hope for the
future is that better techniques of closure will help prevent the occurrence
of tethering in the first place. It will be important for specialized centers to
collaborate to find the answers to these questions.

Scoliosis and Its Management

Scoliosis is an extremely important topic in spina bifida. The condition
may be present at birth (congenital) or develop after birth (paralytic).
Congenital scoliosis is present in around 15 to 25 percent of newborn
babies with spina bifida, most commonly with thoracic lesions and associated vertebral abnormalities. Of more concern to this discussion is paralytic scoliosis, which is usually noted for the first time in school-age children with spina bifida. The condition is common and clearly related to
spinal level: more than 80 percent of children with thoracic spina bifida
develop scoliosis, compared with around 50 percent of those with midlumbar and 20 percent of those with low-lumbar lesions.

Paralytic scoliosis usually has a gradual onset between the ages of five
through nine years, although it may arise for the first time in the second
decade of life. The degree of scoliosis may be stable or progress slowly initially but has the potential to increase rapidly, especially during puberty. A
number of factors, shown in Figure 8.14, have been implicated in the cause
of scoliosis. Certainly, the presence of tethering of the cord and hydromyelia can lead to rapidly progressive scoliosis. Children with asymmetric
muscle function may also be prone to developing scoliosis. The presence
of dislocated hips and pelvic obliquity may be a causal factor as well, for
children make postural adjustments that impose a curve on the spine.

Although mild scoliosis can be quite insignificant to the overall func-

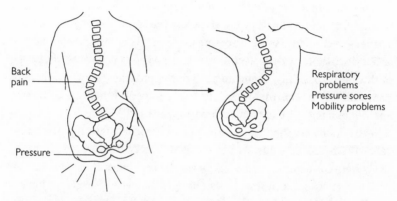

**Risk factors for
progressive scoliosis**

Thoracic lesions
Puberty
Tethering
Hydromyelia
Asymmetric muscle function
Dislocated hip/pelvic obliquity

Back
pain

Pressure

Respiratory
problems
Pressure sores
Mobility problems

Figure 8.14. Paralytic scoliosis in spina bifida may progress rapidly; shown here are some factors that may cause scoliosis to progress.

tion and health of a child, more severe scoliosis can have dire consequences. The development of asymmetric posture, especially in sitting, leads to a dramatic increase in pressure over the ischium (the "sit bone"). Instead of having the body weight evenly distributed over a large sitting area, all the pressure is on one side only. Increasing scoliosis can cause pain and interfere with mobility by making walking more inefficient or even impossible. Scoliosis can also cause back pain. Of most concern is the respiratory compromise that can occur in individuals with very severe scoliosis affecting the thoracic spine. The chest wall can be so misshapen that it dangerously restricts the capacity of the lungs. Such individuals are at risk for pneumonia and are also likely to be poor candidates for anesthesia.

The management of scoliosis aims to preserve symmetry and prevent progression during the vulnerable childhood years. The progression of the curve is monitored closely by the orthopedic surgeon, using clinical assessment and spine X-rays. Geometric techniques are used to measure the degree of curvature precisely. For slowly progressive curves under forty-five degrees, it is generally possible to manage the problem with bracing. Children use lightweight, individually molded orthoses (TLSO, or thoraco-lumbo-sacral orthoses) that can be worn in their chairs or in conjunction with other orthoses (Figure 8.15). These braces are usually not worn while in bed at night to help prevent skin complications.

In many cases, the use of such braces will be sufficient to prevent progression. In others, it allows the child to reach the age of nine to twelve years before surgery is necessary. If the scoliosis is progressing rapidly in spite of this management or if the curve is in excess of forty-five degrees, serious consideration must be given to spinal fusion. Fusing the spine means eliminating further scoliosis across the spine and also preventing further growth of the spine. There are many different surgical approaches, and a discussion of these techniques and methods is beyond the scope of this book. Basically, there are posterior approaches, using permanent hardware such as Harrington rods or Luque rods, and there are combined anterior and posterior (circumferential) approaches (Figure 8.15). It is possible to obtain very significant correction of the scoliosis using these surgical methods. In one study, curves averaging eighty-two degrees preoperatively were corrected to an average of thirty-six degrees after spine fusion. Unfortunately, spine fusion is exceedingly dangerous surgery. There is usually a lot of blood loss, as well as technical difficulties with the instrumentation that is used. There is a risk of further neurologic damage during surgery in the vicinity of the exposed spinal cord. Recovery can be complicated by infections, failure of the instrumentation, and skin breakdown, and the rehabilitation period may be prolonged.

This decision is consequently one of the most frightening that parents have to make. Having weathered so many earlier storms involving their child, parents may find a sense of calm and optimism grow during the early school years, only to be replaced by fear about the prospect of spinal fusion. A trusting partnership between parents and the orthopedic surgeon is essential during this troubled time.

Seizures

Children with neurologic abnormalities are likely to be at increased risk of developing seizures at some time in their lives. Seizures are unpredictable electrical discharges from the brain, usually accompanied by repetitive movements and change or loss of consciousness. Occasionally, the onset of a seizure may herald a shunt problem, such as infection or obstruction. More commonly, however, there is no clear precipitating cause; they just happen. Seizures are more likely to occur in children with shunts, especially those who have had previous shunt infections. About 20–25 percent

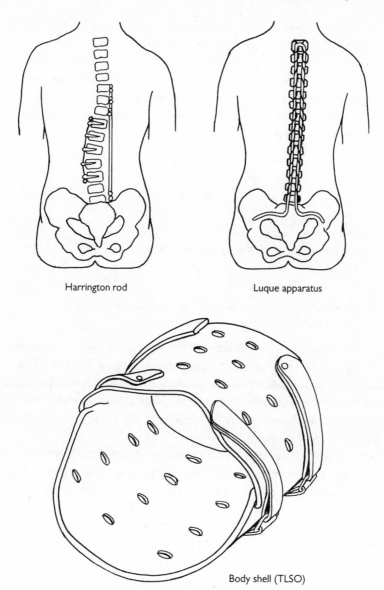

Harrington rod

Luque apparatus

Body shell (TLSO)

Figure 8.15. Management of scoliosis: the TLSO helps prevent progression, but instrumentation and spine fusion are sometimes necessary.

of children with spina bifida develop seizures, although the risk of seizures in those with a history of shunt infections may be doubled.

In many cases, the seizures are grand mal and are frightening experiences for the family. To see a child stiffen, jerk violently, and bite his or her tongue for the first time is terrifying, and common sense about what to do in these circumstances flies out the window. The following steps should be taken to prevent injury:

1. Help the child to the floor or take other measures to prevent falling.
2. Remove sharp objects or other dangers.
3. Turn the child over to one side so that the airway is open in case of vomiting.
4. Loosen clothing around the neck.
5. Do not try to put anything in the child's mouth (a bitten, bleeding tongue will heal quickly).
6. Do not try to restrain the child if he or she is jerking or try to bring the child out of the seizure by shaking him or her or by using any other means.

If the seizure continues for more than five minutes or if one seizure is quickly followed by another, it is advisable to get emergency medical assistance so that medicine can be administered to help bring the seizure under control. If a seizure occurs for the first time, it is very important that the child be evaluated by a neurosurgeon to rule out shunt problems or worsening hydrocephalus.

Although seizures often do not recur, most neurologists recommend the use of an anticonvulsant such as Dilantin to prevent further seizures. In most circumstances, the seizures are fairly easily controlled with a single anticonvulsant medication. If a child who is on anticonvulsant therapy remains seizure free for two or three years, the neurologist may propose to wean her or him off the medicine gradually to see if the child will remain free of seizures. Many times this process is uneventful, and the seizures do not recur. I have known many parents, however, who remain very reluctant to wean their child off anticonvulsants because the possibility of recurrence, even if remote, is so frightening to them.

EMOTIONAL ISSUES

Stress, Coping, and Humor

The early school years can be stressful times for all children, but especially so for a child with a disability who is becoming increasingly aware of her or his differences. The stress may show itself in many ways: irritability, clinginess, or other difficult behavior. These are usually fairly adaptive responses, sending signals to helping adults that all is not well and support is needed. Minor problems and crises are worked through effectively, and the youngsters move on to the next hurdle with a greater sense of self and gradually enhanced self-confidence.

Different children cope with stress in different ways. Some tend to go at the problem like a charging bull at a gate. Others are more timid and tentative, initially withdrawing or responding cautiously. Parents will know their child's temperament well, and they will be the best judges of whether their child's responses are typical or more worrisome. A little stress is helpful and necessary for a growing child, but too much stress can lead to significant anxiety and depression.

Families differ also in their styles of coping with stress, and children learn from their parents in powerful ways. Humor is an especially important way of coping, and I have seen many families for whom humor was second in importance only to their faith.

PARENT-TO-PARENT

"Catherine has needed PT, OT [occupational therapy], speech, and special ed almost without a break over the years. I have learned to take on a new role. I'm not just her mom anymore; I'm her case manager. It's a big responsibility making sure that she is getting the help that she needs. I've learned to be assertive and organized. I don't do a perfect job, but nobody knows her as well as I do!"

"The most important thing for me is to make a point of getting to know the teachers and therapists. Especially at the start of a new year, I try to go to meetings, stop by once or twice after work. If you're going to work as a team, you have to get to know the players."

"Trust your instincts! You know what your child needs! I used to feel so intimidated by all the experts who would talk me out of what I thought was right for Joey, and then time would prove that I was right to start with!"

CHAPTER 9

The Adolescent and Young Adult

Adolescents with chronic conditions are living longer. Almost a third of the individuals with spina bifida in our clinic are thirteen years of age or older. Not only are there important medical issues in this age group, but there also exist unique and critical developmental and psychological issues specific to adolescents and young adults. What services are available to meet these complex needs? Sadly, this age group has historically been neglected when it comes to provision of services. A recent survey from the National Center for Youth with Disabilities (NCYD), an information and resource center in Minneapolis (NCYD, Box 721, University of Minnesota Health Center, 420 Delaware Street, Minneapolis, Minnesota 55455; telephone number [800] 333-6293), showed the continued existence of major service gaps for youth with disabilities such as spina bifida. A large proportion lack access to adequate primary health care. Huge numbers of disabled youngsters are uninsured or lack health care financing. Preventive and health promotion services are variable. Too often there are no services to deal adequately with the complex psychosocial needs of disabled youth. The schools, which are seriously overloaded and underfunded, are left to try to provide needed services. The lack of adequate transportation is a major obstacle to service provision. From an organizational standpoint, the various agencies that are involved, including public health, vocational rehabilitation, social services, and the schools, are often poorly coordinated; as a result, individuals find it difficult or impossible to access available services. Whereas we have committed a lot of our resources to younger children with disabilities, we have left the older ones out in the cold. The tragic consequence is a generation of wasted potential, as we fail to provide the assistance needed for many youngsters to take the next steps toward independence, maturity, and adult fulfillment.

DEVELOPMENTAL ISSUES

Progressions and Expectations

The popular stereotype of adolescence as a sudden explosion of hormones, stress, and family conflict has been greatly exaggerated in recent times. Although hormone surges certainly do occur, adolescence is not all "storm and stress"! Parents, take heart! For most families, these years are challenging yet especially rewarding. This is not the place for advice about parenting a teenager: there are many excellent books on that subject. Just remember that the goal is to teach responsibility and independence. In the early adolescent years, this means clear and consistent limit setting and the establishment of rules and responsibilities. In the later adolescent years, the emphasis shifts to encouraging and supporting young adults in their fledgling efforts to spread their wings. And always, keep the lines of communication open.

Adolescence is really a stepwise maturational process. We are talking about the maturation and unfolding of an adult *person*, not an adult *body*. Puberty is a related but different process, one that is not always in phase with adolescent development. It is possible for a young person to be in midadolescence yet be lacking in pubertal development. In spina bifida, the reverse is frequently true: a thirteen-year-old girl may have a fully mature body, yet she is only beginning to move into early adolescence.

The tasks of adolescence are shown in Figure 9.1. First and foremost, adolescence is about the development of identity, the sense of unique individuality. This task requires some experimentation on the part of the young adolescent, who tries out new identities with different clothes, different ways of talking, different friends. The young person sees how these identities sit with others and modifies them, discards them, and thereby matures.

The process of identity development also requires a separate identity from one's parents. To know who I really am, I have to know who I am not, and that means "I'm not like you, Mom!" Separating from parents, the second task of adolescence, is thus a necessary step in the development of identity. This stage of development hearkens back to the toddler years. The struggle for independence is an ongoing quest about which the adolescent may be quite ambivalent, at times perhaps refusing to join the family on outings or not wanting parents around, and at other times feeling insecure and needing parents' support and help.

The third task of adolescence is the establishment of love and intimacy outside the family. In the next section I will discuss the development of

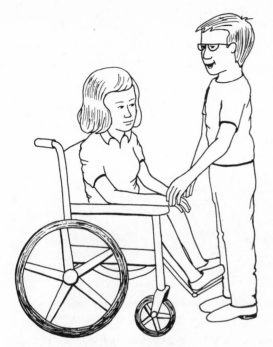

The tasks of adolescence

Developing one's identity

Separating from parents

Learning about love, intimacy, and sexuality

Preparing for the world of work

Figure 9.1. The main developmental tasks of adolescence

sexuality that underlies this task and the special challenges that it poses for adolescents with spina bifida. The fourth major task of adolescence is the development of a vocation, the desire and motivation to study, to earn a living, and to become a self-reliant and productive citizen. Of course, these four broad tasks are interrelated, and their accomplishment to a greater or lesser extent is what being an adult is all about.

Achievement of these developmental tasks can be facilitated by a number of personal attributes and environmental supports (Figure 9.2). In the same way, the presence of a physical disability can alter and interfere with the developmental trajectory of adolescence. It is important to appreciate that it is not so much the disability itself that does this but rather the way in which others respond to the disabled individual and limit his or her ability to make it in the world as an adult.

For example, an overprotected adolescent will perpetually receive reminders, supervision, and help from parents. There will be lower expectations for responsibility and self-reliance. For some parents who are stuck in this pattern of parenting, there may be some deep emotional investment in leaving things the way they are, in providing for their teenager's needs just as they did in earlier years. These are "codependent parents,"

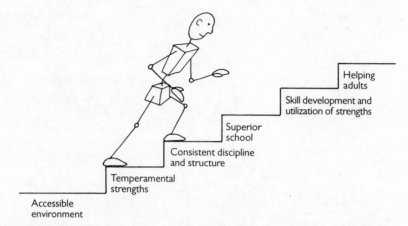

Figure 9.2. Steps toward independence: an adolescent's progress can be helped (or hindered) by many important personal and environmental factors.

who unwittingly help overprotected children become immature and dependent adults.

Another constraint to adolescent development is the social isolation experienced by many adolescents with disabilities. With fewer occasions for socialization with peers, it is harder to make those bonds of identification with a peer group that allow a youngster to pull away from the parents. If such a teenager is not going out to parties and on dates, there will be fewer opportunities for kissing, falling in love, and the other familiar and fumbling steps toward intimacy with another young person.

As we have discussed, identity formation depends on the freedom to experiment with appearances, behaviors, and roles. To hang out with the other kids, an adolescent needs to have some freedom to ride the bus downtown, hang out at the beach, go on an overnight campout, or cruise around the neighborhood. Access to these places for a youngster in a wheelchair may be limited, leading to a lag behind peers in identity development.

The development of identity in adolescence is also inextricably linked with body image, and many youngsters with physical disabilities have some difficulty reconciling their own body images with the perfect, athletic physique that is glorified by the media. There are few, if any, disabled role models for many young adolescents, which hinders their efforts to develop a fuller sense of self.

Finally, finding a vocation and a means to economic independence can be frustrating and hard for a young person who is physically or mentally challenged. Although there has been limited progress in recent years, prejudicial attitudes, limited opportunities, and inadequate supports and services continue to make life difficult for a disabled young adult. Fewer than 20 percent of employment-age people with disabilities are actually employed, and 60–80 percent of such young adults still live with their parents. This situation has to change. One powerful force driving this change is the Americans with Disabilities Act (ADA) of 1991. The potential impact of the ADA will be discussed in Chapter 11.

Sexuality

As young adolescents become increasingly preoccupied with themselves and the changes that are occurring in their bodies, their interest in sex comes to the fore. They may seem quite obsessed with sex and begin the process of dating and early sexual exploration. Although there is great variation in the ages at which different teens go through this, the stages of sexual relationships are pretty similar. Going out on a date, kissing, and petting are typical staging posts in the progression to sexual intimacy.

I have spoken with many adolescents with spina bifida, and it is absolutely clear that all of the above holds true for them. These youngsters are just as interested in sex and just as hungry for knowledge about sexual matters as their peers without spina bifida. Sex education and open communication at home about sex is especially important for these youngsters, because the social isolation to which many of them are subject serves to isolate them from another very important source of information—namely, peers. In a survey we conducted of sexual knowledge among adolescents with spina bifida, it was clear that these teenagers knew less about sex and contraception than other teenagers, and they were less likely to learn about sex from their friends (Sandler et al. 1994). Although the accuracy of talk among peers is certainly open to question, the peer group is a powerful teacher of prevailing attitudes and norms, and this is arguably just as important to a young adolescent in search of sexual identity. It is therefore especially important for educators and parents to teach young adolescents with spina bifida about sex.

Issues of sexuality are also of enormous importance in clinical encounters: it is essential that adolescents understand that it is OK to talk privately with their clinic doctors about their sexual concerns. Of course, sex is not just about bodily sexual functions. Therapeutic efforts need to focus broadly on attitudes, communication, and sexual behavior. I like to ask adolescents in clinic about whether they have been on dates, about crushes, and about steady boyfriends and girlfriends. The problems that they describe are the usual ones that other teenagers have, and the approaches to counseling and anticipatory guidance are not significantly different.

In addition to discussing sexuality for the adolescent age group, we need also to consider the young adult with spina bifida who may be sexually active or about to become sexually active. There are a few myths and misconceptions that may need to be dispelled, but it is my experience that these myths are more often held by medical students and doctors than by the young adults themselves or their parents. For example, it is commonly held that people with spina bifida cannot be sexually active. Interviews with adults with spina bifida provide clear evidence that many, if not most, are indeed sexually active. There are many different sex acts and many ways to achieve sexual gratification and give sexual pleasure to others. The disability may interfere with some of these, but certainly not with all. Nor does it eliminate desire.

Another misconception is that people with spina bifida cannot have babies. Every spina bifida clinic in the country knows of several adult women who have successfully delivered healthy babies and men who have fathered them. It is important to stress the importance of contraception in the clinic setting and to make contraceptive services available when needed. Likewise, the importance of safe sex must be stressed to young adults who are sexually active or likely to become so. One important warning concerns condom use. Latex condoms have the potential to cause severe allergic symptoms in sensitive individuals, and thus the use of polyurethane, tachylon, or "natural" (sheep gut) condoms may be advisable (two of the natural condoms are supposed to be worn to prevent transmission of the virus that causes AIDS).

Until recently, the medical profession tended to steer clear of inquiries about sexuality. Many doctors feel uncomfortable about this area of medicine. Moreover, very limited information exists in the medical literature about sexual function in individuals with spina bifida, which makes it difficult to give sound advice or definite answers to our patients' questions. There has been more research in the area of spinal cord injury, and although some differences are likely, this research helps inform us about sexual function in spina bifida. In our own work with young men with spina bifida, we have found that the majority report that they are able to stimulate erections by masturbation and other techniques of touch (reflex erections). In our research, this was especially likely in those with low-lumbar or sacral lesions. By contrast, few have psychogenic erections (that is, erections from imagining or seeing something "sexy") or spontaneous nocturnal erections. We have actually used a reliable technique of recording penile tumescence and rigidity overnight in a small group of fifteen young men, finding that only two had "normal" nocturnal erections, while seven others had partial erections (Sandler et al. 1996). By inference, it would appear that the individuals with spontaneous erections have "incomplete lesions" of the spinal cord, whereas the majority have "complete lesions." The medical and surgical management options for erection dysfunction have grown in recent years; thus it is possible to obtain erections using papaverine injections (PIPE, or papaverine-induced penile erections), external sheaths and rings, suction devices, or surgical implants (Sloan 1994).

Erections are mediated mainly by the pelvic parasympathetic nerves, whereas ejaculation is mainly a function of the sympathetic nerves. Ejaculation is uncommon in men with spina bifida, although some of the men we interviewed reported ejaculation with orgasm. For others, there may be retrograde ejaculation into the bladder. The use of electrical stimulation may be very effective in producing emission of semen for the purposes of conception. Both men and women with spina bifida in candid interviews have reported pleasurable and climactic sensations with sex, although these may be appreciated in areas of the body other than the genital region.

I believe that others with physical disabilities may be better able to advise young adults about how to prevent or cope with problems that arise with sex. To this end, we have begun to run same-sex groups about sex at a retreat for young adults with spina bifida, where we have an older and more experienced disabled adult as the group facilitator. It is often helpful to remember that sex for people without disabilities is frequently difficult, frustrating, or embarrassing and not the way it appears in the movies! We are all human and we all have something we're embarrassed about. A sense of humor, a simple explanation, an understanding partner, and somebody to ask for advice can all be very helpful.

HABILITATION ISSUES

In this section, we will address issues such as mobility, access, and transportation. Also, the importance of developing independent living skills is stressed.

Mobility

A number of factors make it hard for many adolescents with spina bifida to continue walking as much as they did when they were younger. Increasing obesity may make walking exceedingly tiring. Spinal deformities and contractures of the knees or hips may pose a severe mechanical disadvantage. For some, the occurrence of a fracture or the need for major surgery may cause a prolonged hospitalization, from which they never recover full ambulatory function. About 50 percent of those who are walking with braces at age twelve will have abandoned walking by the age of twenty. This is especially likely for those with lesions at L3 or above. Giving up on walking can be a painful loss for the young adolescent and her or his parents, who all may have invested so much emotionally over the years in the trials and tribulations of walking. In the end, however, one has to be pragmatic, and those who stop walking do so because of the energy expenditure advantages of the wheelchair.

Accessibility

I was talking with a young adult in clinic recently. She was tired of her secretarial job and was in the process of applying to graduate school at a major university. She needed financial aid and had arranged an appointment with the program officer, only to find that the office was on the second floor of an old building that had no wheelchair access and no elevator. How ironic that a program designed to break down barriers actually imposes new ones! Clinicians often take it for granted that patients have fully accessible homes, schools, and workplaces, which often is not the case. Inadequate ramps, temporary classrooms, and insufficient space to maneuver a wheelchair are common problems at school. Even at home, narrow entrances, tight corners, small bathrooms, and other barriers make mobility and transfers difficult or impossible.

Fortunately, the Americans with Disabilities Act is ushering in an era of increasing public accessibility. Lifts are readily available for vans, and are now required on public transportation in the United States. New bus and train stations must be accessible. Wheelchairs on buses need to be secured or fastened to the body of the vehicle, facing forward.

Wheelchair Maintenance

When it comes to choosing among the enormous array of available wheelchairs, young people with spina bifida need to be knowledgeable and sophisticated consumers. Will the chair be used mainly indoors or outdoors? Will it be used during transport in a van or car? Must it fold or dismantle easily for traveling by car? Choices have to be made regarding the frame, the seating, the wheel types, and even the color! Youngsters put great time and effort into the choice of an individualized wheelchair;

moreover, a new chair is likely to cost between two thousand and twenty-eight hundred dollars!

Naturally, it is important to maintain the chair well to get good value from the investment. When we presented a wheelchair maintenance class at a recent young adult retreat, I was very impressed with the expertise of the group in this area. Your local wheelchair distributor and the manufacturer of your chair should provide you with guidelines regarding optimal maintenance.

Driving and Transportation

There is no more powerful and exciting symbol of independence to an American teenager than getting one's own car! For the adolescent with spina bifida, this may pose a few special challenges. The physical needs are really quite easily met with certain modifications, such as hand controls, raised tops, drop floors, and so on. The mental barriers, on the other hand, are more difficult. Poor depth perception, lack of judgment, and other cognitive limitations may truly make driving unsafe. Many parents are good judges as to their teenager's driving potential. If the prospect of driving strikes fear into the hearts of the teenager's parents, their feelings are often justified. It is important to explore this issue and examine the reasons for their fears. If uncertainties remain and expert opinion is needed, driver assessment centers can evaluate the prerequisite skills and provide very helpful information about driving instruction and adaptations. General Motors operates a Mobility Program that can both identify local assessment centers and equipment specialists and offer certain financial breaks for adaptations (call [800] 323-9935). The National Mobility Equipment Dealers Association (NMEDA; call [800] 833-0427) operates a hotline to provide information about the availability of dealers in van conversions, lifts, ramps, and other custom driving equipment.

Enhancing Self-Awareness and Self-Reliance

Studies have repeatedly shown that an individual's employability and independence are not determined by his or her IQ score or the level of spina bifida. Among the most powerful influences on these long-term outcomes is the individual's sense of self. Self-awareness is critically important for the development of self-confidence. When we know our strengths and weaknesses, we develop a realistic and positive outlook. We learn to use our assets to face challenges and gain new skills. Self-awareness leads to self-confidence, and self-confidence leads to self-reliance. Far too many adolescents with spina bifida are lacking in critical skills of self-reliance. About one-third need help with washing, grooming, and hygiene. Most don't know how to plan meals, shop wisely for food, or cook safely. House-keeping and laundry skills are usually inadequate. Few have the skills necessary to manage a bank account or pay the bills. Of course, in their defense, they have often had little exposure to many of these essential in-dependent living skills because of their disabilities. But even in the area of accessing health care, seeking advice, reporting their problems to their doctors, and getting prescriptions filled, many lack the self-reliance that they will need to make it on their own. In one study, only one-third of those young adults with spina bifida and average intelligence could ex-plain anything about what myelomeningocele is. In the clinic, I conduct my clinical interview with the adolescent alone, and I frequently ask these young people what they would say if a friend asks them to explain spina bifida. Few get beyond "It's a hole in the back"! It all starts with self-awareness.

Independent Living Skills Programs

In the United States, a complex maze of community-based services and programs supports individuals with disabilities. There are residential in-dependent living skills programs, day programs, school-based vocational rehabilitation services, group homes, personal care attendants, and so forth. Unfortunately, these services are highly variable and are not orga-nized "under one roof." It can be exceedingly difficult for people to nego-tiate the maze, through all kinds of institutional roadblocks and barriers. Other countries have developed more integrated approaches to providing a necessary range of services. For example, Sweden has community-based "handicapped adult teams" that are responsible for ongoing service co-ordination in health care, habilitation, job training, housing, and welfare.

There are many exciting and innovative programs in this country that focus on the development of independent living skills for older adoles-cents and young adults. Information about these programs can be ob-tained from the SBAA. Among the programs that have come to my at-tention are the Gateway Program in Pittsburgh, the Transition to Adult Living Project at Yale (in New Haven, Connecticut), and the Shepherd's Program about Real Experiences (SPARX) in Atlanta. Successful programs of this type may focus primarily on teaching participants independent living skills while providing important group support as the young people take critical steps toward independence. For example, the adolescents may be enrolled in a kind of "camp" experience, through which they have community outings, access community resources, and engage in problem-solving activities. They may be active learners in a curriculum involving health education, fitness, nutrition, and sexuality. There may be an emphasis on vocational planning and counseling and supervised opportunities to visit and participate in different workplaces. To assist the adolescent in making the transition from the parents' home to independent living, transitional living arrangements may be available, such as supervised, accessible apartments and group homes. Here, the adolescent may receive guidance in shopping, cooking, housekeeping, and financial management. Continuing group support is an important ingredient, as young adults face new, threatening situations. Successful programs also recognize that parents need help and support in managing this transition.

MEDICAL ISSUES

Transition to Adult Health Care Services

Around 90 percent of babies with spina bifida survive into adulthood, which presents a special challenge to health care providers oriented toward pediatrics. Approximately 25 percent of our multidisciplinary clinic population is over sixteen years of age, and other clinics around the country are in a similar situation. It just doesn't make sense for me, a pediatrician, to be examining a twenty-eight-year-old married woman in a pediatric clinic with pink elephants and balloons painted on the walls!

Of course, many of the medical issues of childhood continue to apply in this age group. More important, however, many unique issues exist, and these need to be adequately addressed through adult-oriented health care services. The majority of young adults attending multidisciplinary clinics in this country look to the clinic to provide primary care. If the clinic intends to assume a primary health care role, this must include preventive services such as tetanus boosters and other immunizations. Family planning services and Pap smears should also be readily available. Shunt problems and spinal cord–related symptoms may account for deteriorating health in the young adult, and such conditions may be preventable if spotted early in their course. There are also important health education, vocational, and psychological issues that are specific to this age group.

It is clear that we have the responsibility to plan for an appropriate transition to adult-oriented health care services for tomorrow's adults with spina bifida. Many child-oriented clinics try to group their patients by age, such that on a given day, the clinic team is seeing older individuals. This is a good start and affords the opportunity to use appropriate models

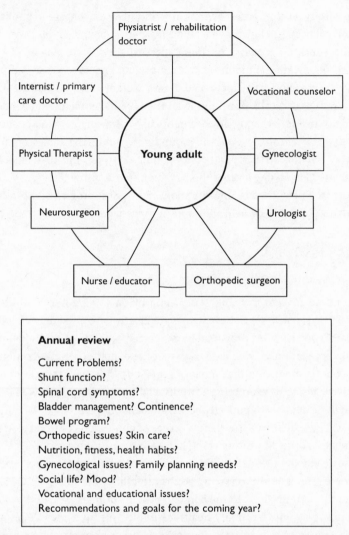

Figure 9.3. The comprehensive health care team for young adults, with key aspects of health care to be addressed in a comprehensive annual review

of care and to provide appropriate health education. The health care team may be broadened to include, for example, an internist, gynecologist, and vocational counselor who are available for consultations. Some clinics have been developed specifically for young adults, providing comprehensive care with in-depth annual review (Figure 9.3). The goal is to assist the young adult in his or her efforts to be healthy, independent, employed, and satisfied and to prevent secondary disabling conditions. These goals are achievable to some extent for all young adults!

Weight Control and Aerobic Exercise

Obesity is a common problem and one that poses a major threat to health. Adults with spina bifida are usually short (the average male is five feet tall and the average female is four feet, six inches) and therefore tend to show excess weight more obviously than most other people. Moreover, the harmful effects of carrying around too much weight are compounded by spinal deformities and small chests that often accompany thoracic spina bifida. In adolescents with limited respiratory reserve, it doesn't take much to tip them into severe respiratory disease. Being substantially overweight and out of condition greatly increases the risk of these life-threatening problems. I recently saw a young teenager who had gained far too much weight during the past few years. He has thoracic spina bifida and a very small chest, and his lung capacity is therefore restricted. He developed bronchitis and pneumonia and had acute respiratory failure, which required intensive care in hospital and dependence on oxygen at home following this hospitalization. After beginning a program of supervised weight control and aerobic exercise, he rapidly lost weight. As his cardiovascular fitness improved, he no longer needed the oxygen. In addition, I am sure that he will be far more likely to withstand the next respiratory infection that comes his way.

Obesity is associated with other health problems as well. Some of these, like hypertension, can be dangerous, whereas others, such as skin infections (intertrigo), are chronic annoyances. Obesity also has the potential to interfere with self-care, personal hygiene, mobility, and participation in some recreational activities.

Adolescents with spina bifida often have low self-concept about their physical appearance. Obesity adds to this burden, and they certainly don't need another reason to feel ashamed. For this reason alone I stress the importance of diet and exercise. It is important for families to understand that caloric needs of youngsters with spina bifida are usually lower than those of people of similar age but without spina bifida. This knowledge alone is not likely to be enough, however. Efforts to lose weight are frequently unsuccessful because the same high-calorie foods are coming home from the grocery store, and there is not sufficient support and reinforcement for losing weight. A weight loss program is greatly enhanced by the use of "the buddy system," in which a peer or a family member is also trying to lose weight. The two offer each other encouragement, advice, and mutual positive feedback as they shed the excess pounds!

Opportunities for sustained aerobic exercise are not always easy to find for young adults with disabilities. Wheeling on exercise tracks and the use of other adaptive exercise equipment may be helpful. Videotapes for wheelchair aerobics are commercially available, such as Richard Simmons's *Reach for Fitness* (Reach Foundation).

Prevention of Osteoporosis

Inactivity leads to osteoporosis, or brittle bones. Bones are a living organ, and there occurs a constant process of bone formation and remodeling. Calcium and minerals are laid down in an organized matrix that makes bones strong. This process is affected by the food we eat (calcium and vitamin D), by our hormones (estrogen), by activity and weight bearing, and by genetic factors. If we look at bone density studies in individuals with spina bifida, the bones are clearly deficient in calcium and minerals. Bones that are lacking in such minerals are prone to fractures. Sometimes we see severe leg fractures in patients who have no recollection of falling or sustaining any trauma. For adolescents and young adults with spina bifida, osteoporosis is especially likely to occur if they are immobilized for long periods because of surgery or if they decide to give up walking.

Fortunately, there are a few things that can be done to help prevent osteoporosis (Figure 9.4). Eating a diet with plenty of vitamin D and calcium is important (skim milk, low-fat yogurt, and calcium-enriched orange juice are good sources). Exposure to sunlight helps provide us with the active form of vitamin D. Therapeutic standing in braces for at least fifteen minutes each day is probably helpful for those who are using wheelchairs exclusively for mobility. For some women, there may also be benefits in taking hormonal supplements in the form of the oral contraception pill. Much research is currently being conducted on osteoporosis prevention. Hopefully, in the years to come, we will know more precisely how to prevent this problem in susceptible people.

Shunt Problems and Chiari Symptoms

Shunt failure is not rare in adolescents and adults. The valve systems may deteriorate over time, failing to regulate CSF pressures consistently. More common, the growth that occurs with puberty may in effect pull the shunt tubing up and out of the abdominal cavity, so that the shunt does not drain normally or becomes obstructed. When shunt problems occur, they may take many forms and become apparent in different ways. The

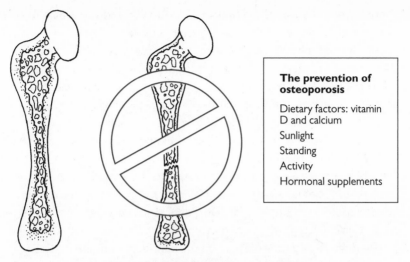

The prevention of osteoporosis

Dietary factors: vitamin D and calcium

Sunlight

Standing

Activity

Hormonal supplements

Figure 9.4. Inactivity leads to brittle bones that fracture easily. Also shown are some factors that are important in preventing osteoporosis.

onset of hydrocephalus may be acute, with severe headache, vomiting, lethargy, and change of consciousness, but it may be far more insidious, characterized by difficulty concentrating, intermittent headaches, sleepiness, or mood changes.

If these subtle changes have occurred, it is important for doctors to investigate the shunt function. A shunt series is a series of plain X-rays which show the shunt and its tubing over its entire length and which enable the doctors to check that the shunt is intact, in the right position, and sufficiently long. The shunt series may show disconnection of the shunt system, or it may show that a young person has "outgrown" the shunt—that is, the shunt tubing is too short. An unenhanced CT scan is the usual technique to establish whether there has been an increase in hydrocephalus. If the ventricles are obviously larger than they were previously, this would be consistent with shunt failure and would require shunt revision. If there are no previous studies with which to compare the CT or if some uncertainty exists about whether the shunt is functioning as it should, the neurosurgeon may elect to tap the shunt. This involves inserting a needle under sterile conditions into the shunt system to examine pressure and flow of CSF. If these investigations suggest shunt malfunction, the neurosurgeon may recommend shunt revision.

One of the problems that commonly arises is the asymptomatic shunt disconnection. A substantial proportion of adolescents with shunts are found on routine examination or shunt series to have a disconnected shunt—that is, a gap or disconnection exists in the shunt tubing (most often in the scalp or neck). The adolescent is unaware of this and exhibits no symptoms to suggest a problem. A CT scan shows no change in ventricle size. We usually assume that the shunt is still draining across the disconnected space or that the youngster is no longer shunt dependent. Some neurosurgeons decide to leave well enough alone and to watch for any signs of deterioration or increasing hydrocephalus. Others feel that there is a substantial risk of sudden, increasing hydrocephalus and that the shunt has to be revised.

Chiari malformation may occasionally cause symptoms in this age group, and the doctor has to be watchful for increasing cranial nerve dysfunction (for example, swallowing difficulties, gagging), dizziness, unsteady gait, neck pain, or weakness in the arms. Chiari symptoms such as these usually indicate pressure on the brainstem associated with shunt malfunction, and they should be investigated as just discussed. It is usually the case that these symptoms resolve themselves after successful shunt revision or posterior cervical decompression.

Spinal Cord Problems

CSF passes from the ventricles into the narrow central canal of the spinal cord. With raised intracranial pressure, the central canal can become dilated, in effect developing a fluid-filled cyst in the spinal cord. This swelling is called hydromyelia (water in the spine) and is fairly common in young adults with spina bifida (Figure 9.5).

Usually, hydromyelia is an incidental finding and does not cause symptoms (McEnery et al. 1992). But hydromyelia may be found in association with rapidly progressive scoliosis, weakness, and increasing tightness in the legs. The neurosurgeon must determine whether the shunt is working normally, for hydromyelia may be caused by inadequately treated hydrocephalus. If hydromyelia symptoms persist despite a functioning shunt, the surgeon may need to place a special shunt to drain fluid from the spinal cord.

Bladder or Kidney Stones

One of the reasons for continuing to monitor the urinary tract with periodic urine checks and ultrasounds is the detection of stones. Stones can form in the bladder or in the kidneys and can develop in the setting of chronic urinary tract infection. They are especially likely to occur in people with augmented bladders. Stones in people with spina bifida are usually painless. One of the tip-offs that there may be a stone is the pres-

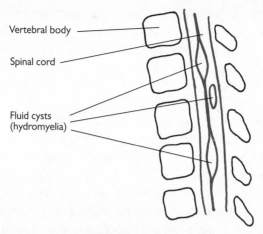

Vertebral body

Spinal cord

Fluid cysts
(hydromyelia)

Figure 9.5. Cysts of fluid in the spinal cord
(hydromyelia) are fairly common in young adults
and can cause rapidly progressing scoliosis and
neurologic changes in the legs.

ence of blood in the urine. Another is the recurrence of bacteriuria after
treatment in a person who does not typically have urinary tract infections. Stones are usually evident on ultrasound examination. Once a stone
is diagnosed, it is important to determine if it is doing any harm, such as
causing troublesome infections or obstructing the kidneys. The urologist
may recommend lithotripsy, which is the use of underwater shock waves
to shatter the stones and make them easier to pass.

Hypertension and Renal Insufficiency

Most adults with spina bifida can look forward to a long life with functioning kidneys. Like most organs of the body, the kidney has much functional reserve; it is therefore possible to get by quite adequately on only a
small percentage of normal kidney tissue. In other words, although many
children have significant reflux and hydronephrosis, they generally have
more than enough good remaining kidney and do not develop signs of
renal insufficiency. Unfortunately, some young adults who have repeated,
severe kidney insults may not have much functional reserve. Thus it is
important to monitor renal function to pick up early signs of renal insufficiency. Among the signs to watch is elevated blood pressure, or hypertension. Although there are many causes of hypertension, the presence of
hypertension in a person with spina bifida raises a suspicion that kidney
function is deteriorating. It is also helpful to check serum creatinine peri-

odically. The first line of therapy for people with hypertension is to lose weight, to exercise, and to restrict salt intake. If these measures are not sufficient, your internist or family physician may recommend antihypertensive medication.

Skin Injury and Pressure Sores

The most underrated organ in our bodies is the skin! Young people with spina bifida have to be constantly vigilant for skin injury. Even as I write, one young man I know is in hospital following a complicated operation to close an enormous pressure sore. Previously, he had developed a sore so large and so deep that it actually eroded into his rectum and necessitated placement of a colostomy. A young woman who had very recently moved away from home into her own apartment developed a pressure sore while standing at a new job and felt compelled temporarily to shelve her independent living plans as a result.

The most common cause of skin injury is pressure from prolonged sitting in one position. This kind of pressure sore usually begins as an area of redness just below the buttock, where the "sit bone," or ischial tuberosity, can be easily felt. If the injury affects the tissues under the skin, there may be a "knot" of hard, swollen, or inflamed tissue under the skin. If the injury progresses, a blister may appear on the skin surface as a result of the damaged or dead skin, along with a discharge of blood and pus, which may be evident on clothing. At this stage, the pressure sore may appear as a clean, punched-out hole that can be superficial or deep, depending on the extent of the damage to underlying skin. It is not uncommon for apparently small areas of redness to reveal much more extensive damage to the underlying tissues.

EMOTIONAL ISSUES

Compliance: Whose Problem Is It Anyway?

Anyone who has ever been told to take some new medicine three or four times a day knows that it is not always easy for a responsible adult to do the right thing! A teenager who doesn't exactly share those adult attributes of responsibility and planfulness is likely to find it harder still. One of the problems that I frequently encounter in the clinic involves teenagers being "noncompliant" with their medical treatments. Usually they have stopped taking their Ditropan or other medications, and they have stopped cathing. Parents express their deep frustrations to me, as their efforts to bribe, beg, coerce, and cajole their youngsters back onto the straight and narrow get nowhere! "He just doesn't seem to care anymore!" they tell me.

Most often, this noncompliance is a result of an adolescent identity crisis, with a touch of adolescent rebellion. Young teenagers with disabilities are having a hard time confronting the fact of their disability, and some may try to deny its existence altogether. Having to take pills at school and having to take scheduled bathroom breaks are irritating reminders of their condition. What better way of denying it than giving up on the treatments? Another powerful factor that comes into play concerns the "ownership" of the disability. As younger children, these kids are used to having their parents give them their medicines, administer their treatments, and perform their catheterizations. It almost feels as if the spina bifida belongs to their parents and the children are just lending their bodies! Then along comes adolescence, a time for asserting one's own identity and separating from one's parents, a time to refuse to do those things that parents bug their teenagers about—cleaning one's room, making the bed, and following the bowel program and doing caths!

The most serious medical consequences of such noncompliance are usually incontinence and constipation, although there can be more significant problems in those youngsters with high-risk urinary tracts. It is important for teenagers to hear and understand that the spina bifida is *their* problem, not the parents' problem, and that ultimately they themselves must take responsibility. Organizational cues, incentives, and negative consequences can all be employed systematically. Sometimes it is necessary to refer a noncompliant youngster for counseling regarding the underlying troubling questions of identity and self-concept.

Adjustment Problems: Confronting Disability

Adolescence is a difficult period of transition, and many young people have trouble adjusting to the changing demands and circumstances of these years. Additional stresses associated with having a disability—or other family and environmental stresses—may lead to temporary changes in mood and behavior. Some teens may become unusually irritable, angry, or defiant. There may be reports of acting out at school or withdrawal from social activities. Problems of this sort are very common and often pass spontaneously or with love and support. Keeping lines of communication open during early adolescence is essential. As a general rule, if problems persist and you, as parents, are worried about them, it is a good idea to consult your doctor, a psychologist, the school guidance counselor, or a mental health professional.

Learned Helplessness

Children who have had things done for them, rather than doing for themselves, are likely to be substantially delayed in the quest for independence that characterizes adolescence. I see many young teenagers with spina bifida who request assistance for everything, including self-help skills, schoolwork, and commonsense, daily problem solving. It is very frustrating for their parents and teachers, who know that they have the skills but are just not in the habit of using these skills independently. Such children seem to lack some problem-solving strategies that come naturally to others. This "learned helplessness" and its accompanying "fear of failure" can prove to be significant barriers to greater independence. One of the most effective interventions that I know is camp or some other similar experience in which the young person leaves home and her or his watchful, attentive parents for a few days and has fun with others of a similar age. An opportunity to see what others do for themselves or a brief heart-to-heart with a camp counselor can turn the young person on to the fun of trying something new by oneself.

Depression

Around 5 to 10 percent of all adolescents get significantly depressed at some time during these years. We are not talking here about feeling sad once in a while but about having a persistent mood change, often accompanied by other symptoms of depression, such as sleep disturbance, loss of concentration, and withdrawal from people and activities. The percentage is higher among young people with disabilities. Depression has a large familial incidence, so that the risk is likely to be much higher if there is a strong family history of depression. It is important for parents, school personnel, and clinicians to be mindful of depression as they evaluate young people with spina bifida. The treatment of depression has come a long way in recent years, both in terms of the availability of therapists experienced in short-term supportive psychotherapy and in terms of the newer medications that are proving to be relatively effective and safe.

PARENT-TO-PARENT

"One of the most difficult aspects of having a child with spina bifida was that I never had heard of it and there were no support groups. Of course, this was nearly twenty years ago. Benjamin's prognosis was not good. The doctors said he would never live, and if he did, he would be a blob in a bed.

Benjamin is now almost twenty years old and will be entering his second year of college in August. He has achieved more than most "normal" kids. With God's help, he will continue to be the best he can be each day.

As a family we never dwelled on what Benjamin couldn't do but on what he could do. He is a child any parent would be proud to have. He has never used his disability as a cop-out but instead to achieve his goals. What a kid!"

"Mike and I have the normal brother-sister relationship. We pick on each other, encourage one another, fight with each other, and love each other. He is a very special person, and I am proud to be his sister. He has achieved much in his life, and I rarely think of him as a 'handicapped' person. Never would I park in a handicapped parking space. Mike can walk like everyone else, and he could use the exercise! My family has never let Mike use spina bifida as a crutch to lean on. He can think for himself and take care of himself. I look forward to the achievements that are yet to come in Mike's life.

Basically, Mike is as 'normal' as the next guy. He is physically challenged, and I must say he deals with the challenge very well. We are all disabled in one way or another . . . in Mike's case you just happen to be able to see his disability."

"Our home is like most homes with a thirteen-year-old teenager, with me constantly saying, 'Turn that music down!' and 'Have you finished your homework?' and 'Go in your room and pick up your clothes!' I smile at myself when I say these things because it was not so long ago that I thought I would never have your typical, everyday things go on in my home. Little did I know how much love and happiness Jonathan could bring into our lives. He continues to teach us the true meaning of love and how to enjoy life to its fullest."

CHAPTER 10

Focus on the Family

FAMILY-CENTERED CARE

One of the major revolutions in children's health care during the last century is the discovery of the critical role of the family in children's lives. It seems laughable that the medical community could have overlooked this simple fact, but it's true! As recently as the 1960s, many major pediatric hospitals had no place for parents to stay with their sick children, and many infants and toddlers literally withered away in the despair of separation. The past ten years have witnessed the most significant commitment to family-centered health care. This trend has been championed by the Association for the Care of Children's Health. In one of their publications (Shelton, Jeppson, and Johnson 1987), the following tenets of family-centered care were laid out:

- Recognizing the family as the constant in children's lives
- Facilitating parent-professional collaboration
- Recognizing and respecting family diversity
- Recognizing unique family strengths and coping methods
- Sharing information fully and continuously
- Encouraging and facilitating family support and family-to-family contact
- Being sensitive to and responding to the family's developmental needs and concerns
- Providing emotional support to families
- Responding to the family's financial needs
- Designing flexible delivery of health care

In my work with children with special needs, I have come to rely on parents as experts on the subject of their children. For example, studies have shown that parents are accurate in estimating their child's level of development (more accurate, in fact, than the child's primary health care provider). This book is written in the spirit of family-centered health care, and this chapter addresses some key family issues.

THE THREE R'S: ROLES, RELATIONSHIPS, AND RESPONSIBILITIES

Some may think that the arrival into a family of a child with special needs changes that family profoundly. Romantics like to portray members of such families as saints who can do no wrong. Skeptics seek psychopathology, offering stereotyped stories of overprotective, enmeshed mothers, interfering in-laws, isolated and rejected husbands, and angry siblings. Such caricatures do little to shed light on the reality of such families. Well, here is the startling truth! About 10 percent of American families include a child with special needs, and the overwhelming majority of these families are ordinary families! Just like yours and mine, they make mistakes, win some important battles, lose others, and strive to do better. They go through some predictable transitions and experience some unpredictable stresses. They cope.

I've known many families of children with spina bifida, and I have a hard time trying to characterize them in any meaningful way. The first thing to stress is that the family is a system in which its members play certain roles and are tied to one another with different relationships. The system is in unique and delicate balance, with any significant change in one part (Dad loses his job and becomes depressed) affecting other parts (Mom takes a part-time job, older son spends more time with Dad and becomes more of a helper at home, younger son feels unhappy and his schoolwork suffers). Family systems may be traditional or nontraditional. There are many diverse, nontraditional families of children with spina bifida, ones whose strengths and coping resources often amaze me. One such family consists of Sherelle, a two-year-old with spina bifida; her young, single mother, who never misses an appointment; and her grandmother, who provides encouragement without taking over responsibility. Other families that come to mind include eight-year-old Dana, with her mother and stepfather, and six-year-old Josh, who comes to clinic with his mother and his stepmother, who are both central figures in his life and who have an exceptionally cooperative relationship with regard to his care.

The next point to stress is the important influence of the family on the ultimate outcome of the child with a disability. I have seen too many examples of this to believe that we are entirely the product of our genes.

Child as baby, princess
Mother as protector, friend, coconspirator, victim
Father as breadwinner, disciplinarian, playmate, part-time supervisor
Older sister as nurse, caretaker, organizer
Younger brother as troublemaker, bad kid

Figure 10.1. Examples of the roles people play in families that may lead to personal stress and family problems

One young man I know has a very significant physical and mental disability, yet his hardworking family has instilled in him a determination, self-reliance, and unconquerable spirit that make me feel very confident he will fulfill his potential in a way that few of us do. Another young man of similar age had low-sacral spina bifida and no hydrocephalus and by all objective criteria has very mild impairments, but years of neglect, abuse, and instability have taken their toll on his self-esteem and capacity to make it as a successful young adult.

Because we recognize the enormous importance of families, we try to understand the *roles* of various family members when we meet them in clinic. Our team has a social worker who is instrumental in this area. Sometimes it can be helpful to talk with families about our hunches and observations by commenting, "You seem to be the decision maker in your family" or "Is it your job in the family to provide all the discipline?" In this way we validate our impressions and also encourage people to think about their families and the roles they play within them. Are these roles appropriate? Is this a role that should be shared more equally? Am I comfortable with playing this role? Some roles are adaptive and make a lot of sense given the unique circumstances of the family. Others may have been adaptive and sensible some time ago but have outlived their usefulness and may even be a barrier to the growth and development of the family. A piece of advice to families is to pay attention to the roles we play, to get rid of old roles that are no longer useful, and to take on one or two new roles that will help the family to move forward in a positive direction. Among the roles that we commonly encounter are those given in Figure 10.1.

Another crucial issue to pay attention to are the *relationships* in the family. Relationships are built on effective communication. When relationships are tense, difficult, or distant, the chances are that a pattern of ineffective or destructive communication has been established. The good news is that these patterns can to a large degree be unlearned and replaced by new communication skills. Instead of talking at other family members, we can learn to be better listeners. Instead of keeping our hurt feelings bottled up inside, we can learn how to assert ourselves in constructive ways. Instead of blaming, we can learn to give clear "I" messages. These and other communication skills are valuable assets for all families, but especially for those under stress.

The last of my three R's is *responsibilities*. We take on many important responsibilities in our families. Some are absolutely basic and essential, such as providing shelter, warmth, food, and security. Sadly, harsh economic realities make even these responsibilities hard to meet for many families at times. This is especially true for families facing enormous and crippling health care costs. I will return to financial issues in the section on money matters later in this chapter. There are other responsibilities that are particularly important for families of children with spina bifida and other disabilities. One of these is the responsibility to overcome family isolation. Some families tend to withdraw socially, to keep to themselves, to the detriment of the disabled child and other family members. Such families must make special efforts to visit others, to belong to churches and other social groups, and in other ways to help build bridges between themselves and their community. Families with a special needs child also have a particular responsibility to celebrate their successes, their small victories, and every display of competence. There is a lot in all our lives to be proud of, and it is so important for family members to develop a sense of family competence. There is nothing wrong with a bit of mutual appreciation to give a boost to family self-esteem!

Another essential responsibility for all families, but especially for those with a disabled child, is to seek help when you need it. No prizes are given for suffering in silence if doing so leaves a difficult situation spiraling out of control. Power struggles, alcoholism, anger, and depression can destroy a family. Although a very troubling family situation cannot be made perfect, steps can be taken to improve things, and one of the first steps is to seek help. Resources may be scarce, but help is usually to be found. One adolescent boy named BJ stopped cathing, started failing at school, and gained a lot of weight. His mother and stepfather brought it to my attention in clinic. BJ was clearly depressed and in need of help. His mother was obviously very frustrated with him, having tried everything to get him back on track, and she was certainly angry with her husband for not supporting her in her efforts to provide structure and discipline. In her frustration, she was becoming increasingly negative and punitive with the boy, and the stepfather was feeling very isolated. Although BJ was the identified patient, the problem went beyond BJ. The family appropriately sought counseling for BJ and accepted suggestions that they also needed to work on consistent parenting strategies and to examine their own relationship. After a few sessions with a social worker, this family was functioning more smoothly, and BJ had resumed his self-care.

I would add that physicians have a responsibility as well in this regard. We need to be sensitive to the stresses that our families feel and to look for evidence of family dysfunction. If we become aware of a problem, it is our responsibility to suggest tactfully that there appears to be a problem and to try to empower the family to do something about it. Not infrequently, these efforts to encourage change are unsuccessful because the family is too entrenched in enabling a pattern of dysfunctional behavior or the family doesn't see the behavior as a problem. There are also occasions when we clinicians have the duty to protect a child from some harm in the family environment (even against the wishes of the family) by contacting the agency responsible for protective services.

MOTHERS AND FATHERS: PARENTAL ADVOCACY

Studies have repeatedly shown that parents of children with such disabilities as spina bifida encounter significant parenting stress. This is especially true at certain times, such as around the time of diagnosis (or birth, in the case of spina bifida), school entry, and adolescence. The burden of stress is carried largely by mothers, even in this relatively enlightened age of shared duty and househusbands! Fathers are often able to insulate themselves from some of the direct effects of the stress through involvement in work and other responsibilities. The level of stress is not directly proportional to some objective measure of the severity of disability. The mother of one quite severely disabled little boy with multiple congenital anomalies is as calm and relaxed as a yoga guru! By contrast, I know a man who has suffered severe grief for years because his son has attention deficit and a learning disability.

It is also clear that parents of children with spina bifida cope admirably with this heightened stress. In fact, the rates of clinical levels of anxiety and depression in such mothers and fathers are not significantly higher than in other mothers and fathers. Perhaps having a baby with special needs brings out some internal coping resources that they did not know they had. Others learn to utilize and depend on family, community, and spiritual resources more than before. For some parents, without doubt, this experience provides a clear purpose in life and brings their parenting responsibilities into sharper focus.

A word here about fathers. A lot of fathers report feeling left out of the whole "parenting thing." They feel that their traditional roles as supporters, breadwinners, and takers out of trash are not sufficient. Times have changed for the role of the father in contemporary American society. With so many working mothers, fathers are sharing a lot of the responsibilities of parenthood. The overwhelming majority are very comfortable taking on this new role. Research on infants and parents shows that fathers are very competent at "reading" their infants and responding with nurturance and parenting skill.

For many fathers, the birth of a baby with spina bifida or other chronic disabling conditions presents a difficult role dilemma. Fathers may feel a powerful need to be stoic—to convey a sense of being in control, of being in charge. Many men also have the role of "Mr. Fix-it" and feel terribly confused when confronted with a situation that cannot be fixed. It is hard for a man who is feeling angry and trying to be stoic and in control of the situation to be on the same wavelength as a grieving wife. Usually, it takes tears, grief, and pain to be really supportive.

My advice to fathers is to make your presence felt as a parent. Let nobody doubt your involvement in issues to do with your children. Attend clinic visits if humanly possible. Even take time off occasionally with your young child to attend sessions with the therapists and early-intervention folk. Don't be ignored! Keep records and stay in touch with therapists and teachers periodically. Express your opinions and ask questions. Have some special time with each of your children individually, to do what they enjoy doing and to pursue "father projects." Follow this advice and you will feel great as a parent and avoid the cycle of disappointment, frustration, and withdrawal.

Mothers and, perhaps to a lesser extent, fathers have a biological need to protect their young. Other species can best protect their defenseless little ones with teeth, claws, cunning, and a ferocious show of strength. I have seen some human parents display the latter two quite effectively! We humans have another, even more potent means of protection at our disposal, namely, knowledge. Knowledge and information are power, especially when it comes to protecting and defending the rights of a disabled child. This is the basis of advocacy: it is fundamental and has an ancient, primal origin. Once parents realize this truth, they seize the knowledge like a magic brass ring, holding on tightly for the ride of a lifetime.

Through increased knowledge and greater participation in the arenas of health care, early intervention, education, transition planning, and the like, parents grow as advocates. And as the children grow and become independent, their parents make subtle shifts from the foreground to the background, from the role of defender and protector to that of supporter and cheerleader.

HUSBANDS AND WIVES

Not all families are traditional, involving a husband and wife; but within a traditional family structure, parents must remember that they were lovers before they were parents and that a healthy family system depends on a strong marital relationship. All married couples face difficulties at times, and one might expect that the anxiety, sadness, and stress of having a child with spina bifida would increase marital strain. In fact, there is no good evidence that the birth of child with spina bifida increases the likelihood of divorce. In one longitudinal study (Tew, Payne, and Laurence 1974), 70 percent of couples had satisfactory marriages after the birth of a child, whether the child had spina bifida or not. Eighteen years later, 75 to 80 percent of the couples had good relationships, as judged by an experienced social worker. Several studies have found no difference in divorce rates among couples with a baby with spina bifida from rates for those who do not have a child with spina bifida. Moreover, there is good evidence that many couples are actually brought closer together by the mutual experience of having a disabled child. Interestingly, those whose child is more severely disabled may experience a very positive effect on their marriage.

BROTHERS AND SISTERS

The sibling relationship is an especially important one in the family because it lasts so long and continues to be important into adulthood. Siblings have many shared experiences over the years, pass through the stages of life at similar times, and may even grow old together, long after their parents have passed on. Many parents express concern about the effect that a child with spina bifida may have on other children in the family. Certainly, parents must be sensitive to this issue and strive to minimize negative effects.

Little research exists on siblings of children with disabilities. A few things are clear, however. First, siblings need information. They need to know the facts of their brother's or sister's spina bifida in order to dispel the myths and misconceptions that may take hold of their imaginations. They also need to know how to talk to their friends about spina bifida.

Second, brothers and sisters also have feelings that require acknowledgment. They may feel angry and complain that vacations and outings are more difficult or constrained by their sibling's motor disability. Some may take on too much caretaking responsibility too early in their lives, a situation that can make them feel deep resentment. They may feel embarrassed about some aspect of their sibling's appearance or behavior and guilty about these feelings or about some act of anger and frustration. Many brothers and sisters may worry about the future: Who will take care of him or her? Will this happen to me? Or to my children?

In one survey, nearly half the mothers of children with spina bifida thought that their other children had suffered. Yet about a third felt that the other children had benefited from the experience. Helping out in the family and sharing some of the burdens and joys can lead to positive feelings of being part of a special family. Most siblings adjust to the situation admirably, showing no unusual levels of resentment or jealousy. It is not altogether surprising that many siblings develop compassion, tolerance, and empathy; and when it comes time to choose a career, many gravitate toward the helping professions (Carr 1991).

Resources for siblings include Siblings for Significant Change ([212] 420-0776) and Siblings Information Network ([203] 648-1205).

GRANDPARENTS AND THE EXTENDED FAMILY

The contemporary role of the grandparent is a rich and varied one. No longer is it that of the grand and powerful matriarch or patriarch but more often that of role model, mentor, storyteller, wizard, and provider of indulgent and unconditional love! Being a grandparent may give a middle-aged person a renewed purpose and meaning in life. Most grandparents enter this role at as young an age as forty or fifty, developing close and long-lasting relationships with their grandchildren. In fact, almost 50 percent of grandparents see a grandchild every day!

The fact that I see so many grandparents in clinic clearly indicates that they play central roles in the lives of most children with spina bifida. The birth of a new grandbaby is a major event in the lives of the grandparents, a time filled with anxiety and reawakening of the old parental protective instincts. When a baby is born with spina bifida, one of the first questions on the mind of the younger parent is, "What am I going to say to my parents? How can I tell them?" And the grandparents, when they are told, experience a dual hurt. Not only is there the loss of the perfect grandbaby, but there is also the hurt they feel for their own child, the baby's parent. All this pain may lead to intense denial and anger. It is not uncommon for intergenerational stresses to arise at this time, with feelings of blame, anger, and hurt. It is so important to work through these problems in order for the family members to draw on each other's support.

CULTURE AND ETHNICITY

In this ever-shrinking world, the United States and other developed countries include a rich variety of cultural and ethnic groups, and any consideration of family issues must acknowledge and celebrate this diversity. Health care professionals need to be especially competent culturally to serve clients from different cultures in their geographic area. Different people have different understandings and explanations of health, disability, and chronic illness. Some may see spina bifida as a divine test; others, as bad blood; and still others, as somebody's fault. They may have very different expectations of survival and very different hopes for the future. Members of one family may be devastated to learn that their daughter is "a slow learner" and not a candidate for college, whereas other parents may have no thoughts of college and be quite content with the prospect that their daughter will help out at home and maybe have children of her own one day. Their responses and decisions need to be understood and evaluated against a cultural backdrop that may differ from that of the health care provider. It is very valuable to have some cultural diversity in the clinic team. As health care professionals, we continually have to confront our biases and "isms" as we care for and learn from the families we treat.

LESSONS IN RESILIENCE: FAMILIES BOUNCING BACK

During the past decade, research on the family's adaptations to disability has shown that most families have important strengths and resources that help them bounce back from adversity. These families are able to search for meaning in their child's problems and discover that meaning from time to time. They are able to regain some control over their lives, developing a sense of mastery as they face future challenges. Resilient families tend to

- Balance the disability with other family needs
- Maintain clear family boundaries

- Become competent at communication
- See situations in a positive light
- Maintain family flexibility
- Be committed to the family unit
- Engage actively in coping strategies
- Be well integrated socially
- Develop cooperative relationships with professionals

MONEY MATTERS: BENEFITS, TAXES, AND ESTATE PLANNING

It is commonly said that doctors make lousy financial decisions, and certainly what follows should not be taken as definitive financial advice (especially in light of the fact that tax and insurance regulations can change over time). My intention here is to summarize some of the key financial issues that families of disabled children and young disabled adults in the United States should know. As I researched this area, I became increasingly perplexed and confused with the complex terminology, changing criteria, and illogical rules. Admittedly, money matters are not my strong suit, but I am certain that most people encounter similar difficulties as they try to figure out financial issues. Indeed, research shows that families with a disabled child suffer financially, with lower wages, enormous expenses, and lack of information regarding benefits and entitlements. Parents have frequently expressed some of these financial pressures. In an effort to provide some of the basic information and also to list some important resources for more detailed information, I have included this section.

Social Security Benefits

The Social Security Administration runs two major programs of relevance to people with disabilities: the Supplemental Security Income Program (SSI), and Social Security Disability Insurance (SSDI). SSI is a program for people with disabilities in financial need. Eligibility for benefits is based on an individual's ability to perform age-appropriate activities, such as those of mobility, self-help skills, communication, and so on. Children under eighteen years of age may qualify for assistance if the family's gross annual income is less than around thirty thousand dollars. Those eighteen or over may be eligible if they have little or no personal income, even if their parents have higher incomes. These eligible young adults should also qualify for Medicaid and food stamps. For more information about SSI, call (800) 772-1213 or (800) 288-7185.

SSDI considers the employment status of the applicant's parents. For example, if at least one parent worked and is now disabled, retired, or deceased, the individual with disabilities may be eligible for SSDI benefits. More information can be obtained by calling the SSDI Hotline at (800) 638-6810.

Work Incentive Programs

In the past, one of the great frustrations of the Social Security system was that people always lost their benefits if they started to earn money from a job. Now several work incentive programs permit benefit recipients to work without immediate loss of benefits. For example, Medicaid benefits may continue under Section 1619b. Moreover, disabled young adults may claim Impairment-Related Work Expenses (IRWEs), which may be deducted from their earned income and which allow them to keep on receiving benefits. IRWEs include such expenses as wheelchairs, braces, other adaptive equipment, and even a job coach! As you can imagine, record keeping is incredibly important in order to document these legitimate expenses.

Another program of interest to disabled adults is PASS (Plan for Achieving Self Support). This program is another means of putting aside funds for the purpose of becoming more competitive in the workplace and deducting these funds from earned income in order to retain benefits for a period of time. The National Rehabilitation Information Center (NARIC) can be contacted for more information at (800) 346-2742.

Income Tax

Families of individuals with disabilities in the United States may claim certain deductions and credits that may help to offset substantially the costs of caring for disabled dependents. There is a personal deduction of $2,350 per dependent. If you provide more than 50 percent of the total costs of support of an individual, then that person may be considered a dependent of yours. This support may include food, shelter, education, medical care, recreation, and gifts. Social Security benefits are considered support from the state.

If your child is an adult over eighteen years of age and earns less than $2,350 per year in gross income, he or she is a dependent. If the young adult is a student under the age of twenty-four years, he or she can earn in excess of this amount and still be considered a dependent for tax purposes.

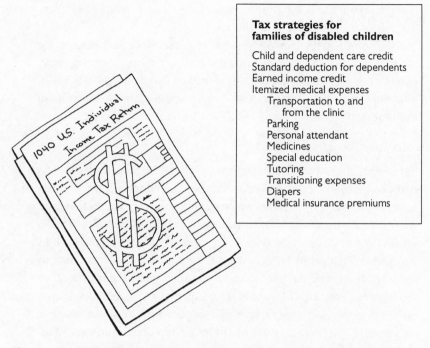

Tax strategies for families of disabled children

Child and dependent care credit
Standard deduction for dependents
Earned income credit
Itemized medical expenses
   Transportation to and
      from the clinic
   Parking
   Personal attendant
   Medicines
   Special education
   Tutoring
   Transitioning expenses
   Diapers
   Medical insurance premiums

Figure 10.2. Medical expenses may be an important deduction on your income taxes. Many costs may qualify as medical expenses for tax purposes.

Your family's medical expenses are deductible if they account for more than 7½ percent of your adjusted gross income. If this is the case, you file using the "long form"—that is, you itemize on Form 1040. Otherwise, you may file on Form 1040A or 1040EZ and take the standard medical expenses deduction. Here, remember that the definition of medical expenses is very broad (see Figure 10.2).

Tax credits are an especially valuable tax strategy because this amount is subtracted directly from the taxes due. The Child and Dependent Care Credit is equal to 20–30 percent of child care expenses up to $2,400 per child (or $4,800 for two or more dependents). Another credit available to those with an income of less than $23,050 is the Earned Income Credit.

Planning sensibly for a disabled child's future is a complex business, including consideration of wills, trusts, and guardianships. More information about taxes and estate planning can be obtained from a tax accountant or by calling Estate Planning for Persons with Disabilities (EPPD) at (800) 448-1071.

HEALTH INSURANCE, HEALTH CARE REFORM, AND THE FAMILY

Heath care reform is a hot topic, and despite the concerns of the American Medical Association, most primary care doctors, including pediatricians, are delighted to see it so high on the national agenda. Unfortunately, as soon as you write anything about health care reform in the United States, it is already out-of-date!

As of 1992, 88 percent of children with chronic illnesses and/or disabilities had some form of health insurance (most of these had private insurance, and about 14 percent had Medicaid). The problem is that the other 12 percent were completely uninsured, meaning their medical needs often go unmet. This figure was as high as 20 percent for Hispanic children. And the proportion of children uninsured overall has grown since 1992.

In most states there is a separately administered program providing health insurance to children under twenty-one years of age with congenital conditions or chronic illnesses. In North Carolina this program is known as Children's Special Health Services and is administered through the Department of the Environment, Health, and Natural Resources. Diagnostic and other comprehensive services are provided free of charge to families who meet financial eligibility criteria.

Medicaid is a federal assistance program. Eligibility is based on income and the category of the individual's condition. Medicaid provides inpatient and outpatient medical care, home health services, dental care, lab costs, X-rays, mental health services, and prescription drugs. Most recipients of SSI are eligible for Medicaid.

President Clinton's health security proposal focused on insurance coverage for all. This proposal and others like it had the potential to improve health care vastly for people with disabilities by providing a federally guaranteed right to care regardless of preexisting conditions. However, the small print revealed concerns that are worth mentioning. There were exclusions for durable medical equipment; in other words, certain braces and customized medical equipment would likely not have been covered by this plan. There may have been major limitations for outpatient rehabilitation services, including therapy to maintain existing levels of function. I wonder about the extent to which expensive early-intervention services such as OT/PT and speech and language would have been covered.

This plan was torpedoed by Congress and special interests, and the political focus shifted to balancing the federal budget and cutting entitlement programs. Legislation threatens funds that provide essential health services to women and children. In North Carolina alone, the proposed cuts in the Maternal and Child Health Block Grant would mean substantial cutbacks in medical care: five thousand fewer low-income children with chronic disabilities and illnesses would receive diagnostic and treatment services. Moreover, the proposed cuts in Medicaid will have far-reaching effects.

Even without health care reform legislation in Washington, the field of health care is changing rapidly as corporatized managed care grows by leaps and bounds. There is a continuum of models of managed care, from primary care case management models, to capitated plans with carve-outs for special populations, to fully capitated systems with special rates for those with disabilities. Most managed care health plans restrict specialized services and treatments. These plans are consumer-driven, and because the majority of healthy American families want to pay lower monthly premiums, the plans that are offered are more restrictive. Unfortunately, consumers are usually not well informed about the plans, and families with special needs children discover unforeseen restrictions only after they have joined a plan. It is critical for health care providers to advocate for needed services and to help educate families to make appropriate choices among plans.

There is great concern and a feeling of uncertainty about health care and the provision of services for children with special needs in the future. It is vital that those of us involved in this field—as doctors, therapists, parents, and recipients of needed therapy—make our concerns known on Capitol Hill as the health care debate takes shape.

CHAPTER 11

Focus on Education and Work

The ongoing debates about education in the United States have caused us to focus on the many problems facing schools. Violence, poverty, drugs, and declining standards are of great concern and raise enormous public policy issues. Sometimes, in a climate like this, it is easy to forget the positive as we focus on the negative. Indeed, many positive trends exist in American education. In no area is this more true than in the education of children with differences.

Only twenty years ago, almost half of all children with special needs were out of school or inappropriately placed. Typically, they were in self-contained and separate settings; had severe restrictions on activities and educational experiences; and suffered isolation, rejection, and humiliation from their peers. There was a widespread lack of awareness regarding disabilities on the part of teachers and school administrators. Most parents, although unhappy with the system, felt excluded from the process and powerless to effect changes.

Then along came the test case, *Mills v. Washington, D.C., Board of Education*, in which the Supreme Court ruled that lack of money was not an excuse to deny children their rights to an appropriate education. Out of this followed new federal legislation, the 1975 Education for All Handicapped Act (Public Law 94-142), and the 1990 updated legislation, the Individuals with Disabilities Education Act, or IDEA (Public Law 101-476). These laws have revolutionized education for disabled students. Yet limited resources and adversarial relationships persist. With more than three hundred students with disabilities dropping out of school each day, major challenges remain.

Improved detection and tracking systems for children with special needs

Greater access to evaluation and therapy services

Comprehensive programs for children from birth through three years of age

Free, appropriate public education for children aged three to five years

Close involvement of parents in the process of reviewing and planning child's education

Goals and services take account of family strengths and needs

---

Figure 11.1. Benefits of Public Law 99-457 and the Individualized Family Service Plan (IFSP)

Public Law 99-457 and Early Intervention

Fueled by the documented benefits of Headstart, preschool education, and early intervention, Public Law (PL) 99-457 came into being in 1986 (Figure 11.1). This major piece of federal legislation is concerned with early intervention and preschool education for young children with developmental problems or at risk of developmental disability. The legislation recognizes the unique role of the family in intervention and the enormous potential benefits from agencies and service coordinators working in partnership with the family to effect change. Such recognition is embodied in the Individualized Family Service Plan (IFSP), which is a process of review and planning that involves parents, service providers, and coordinators and which sets forth mutual goals for the child, taking account of individual and family strengths and needs.

Under PL 99-457, states have been supported in developing their own systems for determining eligibility for services, early detection (child find) and tracking services, evaluation and therapy, and public awareness campaigns. Part H ensures federal help in planning and implementing comprehensive, interagency programs for the birth-to-three age group and their families. At least forty states have established a coordinated system under Part H. The system of services is supervised by a designated lead agency and a governor-appointed Interagency Coordinating Council. In North Carolina, multidisciplinary evaluations of young children are conducted free of charge to parents at a network of state-funded developmental evaluation centers (DECs). Home-based and center-based services, such as physical therapy, speech and language therapy, and other developmentally appropriate early interventions are available from a variety of centers and agencies, including home health agencies, private therapists, and other early-intervention services. Services are not free but are usually provided on a sliding fee scale.

Part B (or Section 619) of PL 99-457 provides funding incentives to states to develop free, appropriate public education for three- to five-year-old children with disabilities or atypical development. In most states, the lead agency for these services is the public school system. Children with spina bifida qualify for services, including special education, physical therapy, and so on, at age three. Usually, the simplest way into the system is to contact the director of exceptional children's services through administration at the local school to inform her or him about your child's needs. For your child to be served in a developmental preschool class, the schools must typically use some form of categorical label for the purposes of their record keeping. Services may be provided under the specific category. "Other Health Impaired," "Physical Impairment," or the like.

The exciting thing for me as a developmental pediatrician is to see that this system, with its massive bureaucracy and far-reaching effects, actually works! In the past five years, I have noticed a dramatic increase in the number of young children with special needs who are receiving excellent services in infancy and in the preschool years. It is beyond question that the direct therapy, opportunities for structured play, social opportunity and stimulation, and family-centeredness improve outcomes. In addition, families are generally very satisfied with the services provided to their young children. The most pressing problem appears to be the high cost of early-intervention services for infants and toddlers. Such therapy is frequently not covered by insurance, which may cause middle-class families to carry a huge financial burden.

PUBLIC LAWS 94-142 AND 101-476 (IDEA) AND THE INDIVIDUALIZED EDUCATION PLAN (IEP)

PL 94-142, now succeeded by PL 101-476, the Individuals with Disabilities Education Act (IDEA), provides federal money to help reimburse school districts for the extra costs of educating children with disabilities, so long as they comply with a number of important requirements for appropriate placement, notification of parents, impartial hearings, and other aspects of due process. The law is also explicit about the rights of parents with special needs kids and the responsibilities of the schools in providing services.

The laws ensure that all exceptional children must be provided a free, appropriate public education, with provision of special education and related services. When a parent, teacher, or another person thinks that a particular child may need such services, a referral is made to the principal or the superintendent of schools. An evaluation process takes place, which may include formal psychoeducational testing. Alternatively, a team of specialists and teachers in the school, usually known as an Individual Assistance Team or School-Based Committee, may make recommendations regarding appropriate modifications and classroom strategies. If the school-based evaluation is not adequate, the parents have the right to an independent evaluation, which may under some circumstances be paid for by the schools. However, parents will generally need written approval for payment in advance of getting such an independent evaluation.

If the evaluation provides sufficient evidence that a child does need special education and related services, then an IEP must be developed within thirty days. An IEP is a written plan regarding the services needed, developed by parent(s), teacher, and representative(s) from the school system. The school system has to schedule the IEP meeting at a mutually convenient time and place. The IEP must include the following:

- A statement of the child's present educational performance
- A statement of goals for the year and short-term measurable instructional objectives
- A statement of the extent of services to be provided and also the degree to which a child is able to participate in regular education programs

Parents have the right and responsibility to ask for additions, changes, or different priorities in the IEP. They may examine all the relevant records, including those from independent evaluations, and they may invite others to attend the IEP meeting. When appropriate, the child may be included in the IEP meeting as well. The schools have the responsibility to arrange IEP meetings once each year to review the plan and develop a new one for the coming year. Children with special needs are also required to be reevaluated every three years to determine their continued eligibility for services.

For most children with spina bifida, the IEP should include such related services as intermittent catheterization. These services should be specific and include who will be doing the cath and at what times. Transportation needs, physical therapy, occupational therapy, and recreation may all need to be addressed. In addition, the IEP should contain certain self-care goals, which may include aspects of mobility, toileting, dressing, and being appropriately assertive.

To obtain more details about parents' rights under IDEA, contact the
director of exceptional children's services in your county's school system.

WHAT'S SO SPECIAL ABOUT SPECIAL EDUCATION?

When PL 94-142 came into being in 1975, the main thrust of the legislation was to ensure that children with special needs were educated in
the least restrictive environment. Where previously almost all children
with spina bifida would have been restricted to special schools, the 1980s
saw a number of innovations that enabled such children to join their
peers without spina bifida. This was true for children with more common disabilities too, such as learning disabilities and mild mental retardation. Under the impetus of PL 94-142, there was strong commitment
to mainstreaming children with disabilities in regular schools, which was
achieved primarily by relying on a "pull-out" model. For example, a student with significant learning disabilities may have been with his or her
regular peer group for art, PE, and other nonacademic classes but then
pulled out of the classroom for academic instruction. Thus mainstreaming provided many students with opportunities for socializing with the
nondisabled peer group, but in many cases this was overshadowed by the
negative effects of being yanked out to go to the special class, with all
the attendant isolation and stigma. Under this "pull-out" model and with
huge increases in identification of students with disabilities, the field of
special education flourished. Instead of regular teachers learning how to
include children with special needs in the regular class, this responsibility
became the exclusive domain of the special educators.

During the last few years, many parents have questioned the adequacy
of the "pull-out" model. Increasingly, there is an awareness that children
with special needs should be and can be included more in the regular classroom. Many parent groups advocate strongly for "inclusionary
models," and such models are being adopted by schools to ever greater ex-
tents. These models do not do away with special education: regular classroom teachers will depend on those in special education for ideas, educational strategies, and ways to assess progress. Such models of inclusion
have been successfully implemented in many schools and have the potential to enhance the self-esteem of children, both those with and those
without disabilities. To be successful, such classes must maintain positive expectations for success and utilize strengths and abilities rather than
focus on deficits. I have some concerns about the dogmatic pursuit of "full

inclusion," whereby all children, even those with severe disabilities, have their needs met in the regular classroom. It is not that I think it can't work, but I am concerned that to do it right will require a very strong commitment and reallocation of resources. Without such commitment, inclusion may be unfairly used as the justification for pulling the plug on needed services. If this were to happen, inclusion will sadly prove to be an illusion.

PARENT-TEACHER COOPERATION AND SCHOOL ADVOCACY

Last week, I was contacted by a parent because of a litany of concerns about inappropriate and unfair treatment of her child at school. She was angry because her daughter was not allowed enough time between classes, there were no adaptations in PE class, the principal was refusing to meet with her, and so on. On her behalf, I contacted the principal of the school, who expressed a willingness to work with the family. However, he told me, the child's mother had been verbally abusive to his teaching staff and had not shown up at a meeting that she herself had arranged. What a sad state of affairs, and one that regrettably happens far too frequently, to the detriment of a child's education.

Like everything else, parent-teacher relationships and school advocacy are skills that can be enhanced with advice and practice. Also, like any relationship, it takes two to tango; both parents and school personnel have to know their steps in order to dance! Here are some tips for parents to help them develop mutually rewarding interactions with school personnel for the benefit of the child. Some of these tips come from a survey of special education teachers, and some, from parents who have had to learn from their mistakes.

- Work with your child at home on her or his schoolwork.
- Make sure that your child follows through on homework assignments.
- Communicate frequently with teachers.
- Talk to teachers about your child having some assignments over the summer, and keep a folder of work done during the summer.
- Visit the classroom from time to time.
- Show your appreciation of teachers' efforts.
- Keep an organized notebook or file regarding school issues.
- Always write things down or keep items in the appropriate place—for example, keep copies of letters, summarize phone calls, and write down anecdotes or examples.

- Prepare for meetings, such as those for IEPs.
- Consider ahead of time what your goals are for a meeting.
- Try to set up "win-win" situations, where you and the school are working toward the same objective.
- Take the other parent or another supportive person along to important meetings.
- Do not assume an adversarial stance with the school from the start.
- Look for allies in the teaching staff.
- Practice assertiveness without hostility: use empathy and grace.
- Communicate openly, and ask questions.
- If conflict arises, do not involve your child directly: pawns always suffer!
- Try to keep interpersonal issues out of the way; focus instead on the problems and the goals.
- Prioritize; pick your battles.
- Celebrate small victories and successes.

EDUCATION MANAGEMENT STRATEGIES

I see many children with spina bifida who have significant learning problems. These were discussed in some depth in Chapter 8. Working for many years with a skilled multidisciplinary team of developmental specialists, I have come to learn something about strategies that may help a child to overcome or to bypass a learning difficulty. Many of these will be very familiar to teachers, but some of these will be refreshing and novel ideas that may have important implications in the classroom or while studying at home. I offer these here as possibilities for discussion and mutual problem solving between parents and school personnel (Figure 11.2).

TRANSITION PLANNING: HIGH SCHOOL AND BEYOND

Just as school entry poses special challenges, so too does school leaving. Among the challenges for youngsters with disabilities and their parents in the high school years are identifying and developing one's talents so as to begin to define career possibilities. Once a range of career possibilities is decided on, then comes the challenge of pursuing and obtaining the necessary education and training.

The heightened stresses of these years is aggravated by the knowledge that the clock is ticking away and the entitlements to special education and related services are going to end soon (services under IDEA stop at

Classroom management techniques for aiding students who have attention problems

Traditional closed classrooms are preferred (and should be requested) over an open-style classroom that magnifies all auditory and visual distraction.

Preferential seating at the front of the class and close to the speaker should be arranged. Seating away from high-traffic areas (doorways, pencil sharpeners) is desirable.

All extraneous noises and visual stimuli should be minimized, especially when giving instructions and teaching new concepts.

Teachers should always command the child's attention, if necessary by using verbal or physical cues such as lightly touching her or his shoulder or desk or using a "secret" signal. It is important not to embarrass the child.

Directions will be easier for the child to follow if they are given in clear, well-articulated, and simply constructed sentences. Avoid complex or compound sentences.

New information should be separated into small, well-defined sentences.

Talking slowly and frequently restating oral information will aid in comprehension.

Verbal instruction should be accompanied by visual reference (pictures, diagrams, outlines, models) and demonstration.

Because memory is best for real-life events or occurrences, experiential approaches to learning and concrete examples are beneficial.

Periodic feedback should be required from the child to ensure that he or she is listening to the speech message.

Instructions may need to be repeated following each class on an individual basis if the child has not been able to comprehend the material. Encourage the child to repeat what she or he thinks was said. Assignment books are often beneficial.

Move on to new areas of academic instruction gradually, always reviewing past material so that the child can experience some degree of success.

New concepts should be previewed at the beginning of a lesson and highlighted at the end of the lesson. Writing them on the board may also reinforce the student's attention to them.

The teaching process should involve active participation by the student, as opposed to passive listening. Reciprocal teaching techniques in which students assume the role of teacher in small groups will help maintain attention and reinforce comprehension of material.

Seat work and passive listening tasks should be punctuated by breaks or activities that provide opportunity for the student to get up and move about.

Figure 11.2. Education management strategies for children with attention, memory, or visual-perceptual problems

A tape recorder may be helpful in the teaching process. You may opt to record lessons or instructions on tape for the child to review at home.

Take care not to discipline a child when his or her misbehavior or lack of willingness to participate in a group activity or to complete a task may be due to confusion caused by problems with attention.

Encourage the child to ask questions when she or he is confused, praising her or him for such initiative. Establishing a positive feeling about asking questions or asking for repetition is *essential* and will be irreplaceable as the child progresses through school.

Children with attention difficulties are typically fatigued after a full day at school as a result of trying to overcome external distractions and auditory confusion. It may be helpful to plan more difficult lessons for early in the day or to alternate lessons that require greater auditory attention with more visual or independent ones.

Give the child praise and reinforcement for even minimal improvement. Encouragement and support are key factors in developing patterns of success.

All adjustments should be made so as not to draw negative attention to the particular student—that is, do not call the student by name and tell him or her to listen. Avoid public identification, or identify the child in a positive sense: "I like the way [name] is all ready to listen."

Strategies for improving memory in children with memory problems

Rehearsal. Rehearsal is the continuous repetition, either overtly or covertly, of an item, phrase, or sentence. For rehearsal to be effective, it must be deliberate.

Chunking. Chunking is the organization of information into small sets. Words or numbers are more easily remembered if they are arranged and memorized in units of threes or fours.

Elaboration. Elaboration is the incorporation of new information into existing knowledge. The student activates what he or she already knows about a subject and then expands on the new information with new linkages and elaborate embellishment.

Mnemonic devices. Mnemonic devices are formulas or codes used as an aid in remembering. For example, the first letter of the major countries of Western Europe (that is, Spain, Austria, France, England, Germany, and Italy) spell SAFE GI. If the student can remember this phrase, it can serve as an aid in recalling the countries.

Imagery. Imagery is internal mental pictures or images. The association of an item with a mental picture has the property of facilitating recall.

Figure 11.2. (*continued*)

Multisensory stimulation. Multisensory stimulation is the application of two or
more of the senses in learning a task. For example, recall of a written word can
be increased by simultaneously saying, seeing, hearing, and writing the word.

Advanced organizers. Advanced organizers are central ideas or key concepts
around which new information is organized. To master subject matter
efficiently, the student should first be exposed to anchoring ideas around
which new knowledge can be arranged.

Self-testing. Students with memory difficulties should devise methods for testing
themselves. They should be given sample questions. They often have great
difficulty knowing what they know and when they can stop studying. Their
parents and teachers and the students themselves should stress self-testing
behaviors while studying for examinations.

In addition to these techniques, teachers can structure the learning environment
in such a way as to expedite the recall of information. The following actions and
principles will aid the teacher in providing a setting in which efficient and
spontaneous recall is possible:

- Tell the student, beforehand, what to remember.
- Material that is organized is more easily learned than material presented in a
  random fashion.
- Let the student know how the material has been organized.
- Material that has been partially learned is more readily retained than is new
  material.
- Give the student sufficient time to memorize new material.
- Learning sessions should be kept as short as possible, with rest pauses
  provided throughout the entire learning period.
- Provide reinforcement and feedback.
- Consideration should be given to allowing such children to take tests
  untimed, especially standardized entrance examinations. Alternatively, on a
  quiz, children with memory problems should be allowed to solve fewer
  problems or somehow to receive extra time inconspicuously.

Strategies for children with visual-perceptual problems

Games that involve matching shapes, objects, pictures, and letters may improve
spatial organization.

Tasks that emphasize attention to visual details and visual scanning are important.

Tactile aids and multisensory methods may help with learning letters and
numbers.

Figure 11.2. (*continued*)

A reading program that stresses phonetic skills, structural analysis, and language may be most appropriate, rather than flash cards, to build sight-word vocabulary.

Using a card with a window in it may help a child to track across the page while reading.

Using such visual organizers as lined paper, dot-to-dot letter outlines, and graph paper may be helpful.

Children should be encouraged to use verbal mediation strategies, such as "down, up, and around" when they write the letter "b."

The use of manipulatives, number lines, and other sensorimotor techniques should be encouraged in order to teach children number and quantitative concepts. Blocks and Geoboards can also be helpful in understanding part-whole relationships.

Children with arithmetic problems should not be discouraged from using their fingers to count. Older children should be encouraged to use calculators for computation.

Figure 11.2. (*continued*)

age twenty or earlier if the young adult leaves school). This places a much greater burden of responsibility on the family for coordinating the transition to adulthood. Also, there is a growing need for the emerging young adult to practice self-advocacy and self-determination. The skills for self-determination must be taught: they require preparation and practice.

Another complicating factor is that the world after school is inherently more complex. Whereas educational and support services during the school years were all under the one roof of the school system, the young adult is entering a baffling array of service providers, including Social Security, health care, vocational rehabilitation, higher education, and adult training. Each one of these has a different agenda, address, bureaucracy, and eligibility requirements!

Fortunately, IDEA recognized these major hurdles and included provisions for transition planning and services. Unfortunately, these provisions are often not adequately applied, and thus young people get to the end of their school years and suddenly wake up one morning with nothing to do! Planning should begin in high school. *The IEP for disabled students should include transition plans by age sixteen years.* This may take the form of funded training programs for vocational experience, vocational education, and counseling. Other countries, especially the European countries, have done a much better job in this area than has the United States, with extensive partnerships between education and industry to help young adults into positions of gainful employment.

HIGHER EDUCATION AND ADULT TRAINING

At a recent retreat for young adults with spina bifida, I was very impressed with a group of young men and women who were pursuing higher education with great determination. They were candidly discussing some of the challenges and hurdles that they were facing, while full of enthusiasm and a sense of accomplishment. They knew they were taking enormous steps forward in their lives. They offered one another support and also inspired some of the high school students and other young people at the retreat to pursue their dreams. One person offered this piece of advice, which sticks in my mind: "Don't let anyone tell you what you cannot do!"

A few of these people had graduated from or were attending four-year colleges. Many others were at junior or community colleges. In the United States there is an enormous network of community colleges that offer courses leading to a high school diploma, a certificate degree, or an associate's degree. These colleges have low tuition rates and offer a wide range of disability-related support services, including financial aid and vocational rehabilitation.

Further information about higher education can be obtained by calling HEATH (Higher Education and Adult Training for People with Handicaps) at (800) 544-3284 or AHEAD (Association on Higher Education and Disability) at (614) 488-4972. In addition, G. A. Schlachter and R. D. Webb, *Financial Aid for the Disabled and Their Families, 1995–1996* (Redwood City, Calif.: Reference Service Press, 1995), is a useful publication, which may be obtained by calling (415) 594-0743. A copy of "Transition Summary" published by the National Information Center for Children and Youth with Disabilities (NICHCY) may be obtained by calling (800) 695-0285. Those who are interested in a career in science, math, or engineering should contact the American Association for the Advancement of Science (AAAS), which has been a trendsetter in putting disability issues on its agenda. The AAAS, in conjunction with the American Institute for Research, has published two helpful brochures entitled "Find Your Future" and "You're in Charge," which can be ordered by calling (202) 326-6630.

MAKING IT IN THE WORLD OF WORK

Two-thirds of people with disabilities in the United States are not working. Given what we know about how work builds self-concept and contributes to overall life satisfaction, this statistic is startling and demoralizing.

Several different employment options exist for people with disabilities: competitive employment, transitional employment, supported employment, and sheltered employment. Competitive employment refers to jobs in the open labor market. Individuals in competitive employment maintain their jobs without support. Training requirements for different jobs vary but are usually minimal for an enormous variety of entry-level jobs. An individual may need on-the-job training, which is provided by the employer. Transitional employment is a job requiring initial training and support. Typically, the support and follow-up may last for six months, after which time the individual is in effect in a competitive or unsupported employment position.

Supported employment refers to competitive work in integrated settings—that is, regular workplaces with nondisabled fellow workers. The individual may require ongoing support in his or her job. Supported employment options include an individual placement with a job coach available to provide supervision and training, an enclave of disabled workers with a supervisor, or a mobile work crew. Sheltered employment refers to workshops or other work settings where fellow workers are also adults with disabilities.

Making it in the world of work is a stepwise process, and those first steps are the most important. Too often I see young people take one look at an option, reject it, and then look no further. Take the first step and be patient, and it will lead to bigger and better possibilities. Part-time work and temporary work may be valuable first steps. Another option is to work as a volunteer in your community as a stepping-stone to other opportunities. The Peace Corps and VISTA (Volunteers in Service to America) may be helpful resources and can be contacted at (800) 424-8580.

The most important resource is vocational rehabilitation (VR). Each state has a central VR office, and there are local offices in or near most communities. The first step is to make an application for VR services. The application will be assigned to a VR counselor, who will initially work with the applicant to determine whether he or she is eligible. Eligibility is based on the presence of a physical or mental disability that poses a substantial obstacle to employment. There also has to be a reasonable expectation that the applicant will benefit from VR services. Almost every young person with spina bifida should therefore be eligible.

VR covers a range of services that can help a person along the road to employment. Under Section 103(a) of the 1973 Rehabilitation Act, services include evaluation, counseling, medical care, job training, maintenance payments, transportation, aids and devices, tools and equipment, and suitable job placement. VR can help to negotiate with employers regarding "reasonable accommodations" to make the workplace more accessible and usable. Under the terms of the law, employers are required to make structural modifications, such as to ramps, elevators, and parking. They are also required to modify schedules and provide equipment that is necessary for a disabled worker to do his or her job satisfactorily. Further advice regarding access issues at work and reasonable accommodations can be obtained by calling the Access Board at (800) USA-ABLE, or (800) 872-2253; the Job Accommodation Network at (800) JAN-PCEH, or (800) 526-7234; or your local VR office.

The Americans with Disabilities Act (ADA)

The ADA (Public Law 101-336), signed into law by President George Bush in 1990, was landmark legislation in the United States, affecting the lives of some forty-three million Americans with disabilities. In recent years, other countries such as the United Kingdom have also passed disability legislation, but none is as far-reaching as the ADA.

Essentially, the ADA makes it unlawful to discriminate against qualified individuals with a disability. In effect, all individuals with spina bifida who are qualified to perform the essential duties of a job would be protected under the terms of the law. The legislation is very broad in scope, affecting the workplace, accommodation, transportation, and telecommunications. In the area of employment, the law prohibits discrimination in recruitment, hiring, job assignments, pay, training, promotions, and benefits and is very clear about acceptable practices. For example, an employer cannot inquire if a person has a disability and cannot require someone to take medical or other tests that tend to screen out people with disabilities. Employers need to provide "reasonable accommodations" to allow disabled employees to perform the job effectively, although they are not required to do so if that would impose "undue hardship" on business operations. Accommodations may include modifying equipment, adjusting schedules, and making the workplace readily accessible (Figure 11.3).

Many young people ask, "Should I tell my employer that I have a dis-

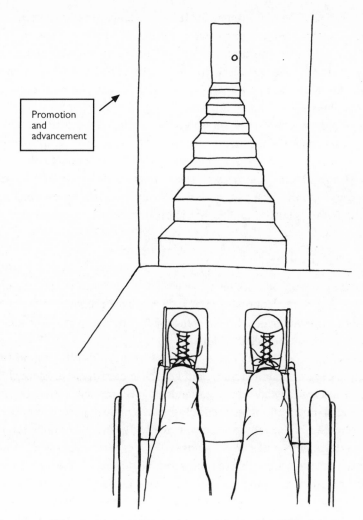

Figure 11.3. The Americans with Disabilities Act (ADA) is potentially far-reaching legislation to protect people with disabilities from discrimination, especially in the workplace.

ability?" If you think you will need some accommodation to get the job or to do it effectively, then you should accurately inform your employer about what you will need. It is your responsibility to tell your employer what your special needs are. It is helpful to know that a tax credit of up to five thousand dollars may be available to small businesses to assist them in complying with your requirements for accessibility.

The terms of the law apply to all employers with fifteen or more employees. The ADA is enforced by the U.S. Equal Employment Opportunity Commission (EEOC) and the U.S. Department of Justice. To protect your rights, it is advisable to contact the EEOC promptly if discrimination is suspected and to file a charge within six months of the alleged discrimination. The EEOC ([202] 663-4900) has a booklet available on your employment rights (1991).

The ADA also addresses transportation rights of the disabled. Public transportation is required to be accessible, as are new construction and building alterations. For more specific information about the way the ADA applies in these areas, the Department of Transportation ([202] 366-9305) and the Architectural and Transportation Barriers Compliance Board ([800] USA-ABLE, or [800] 872-2253) are helpful resources.

FRIENDS AND FRIENDSHIPS

Attending school or working a job provides opportunities for making friends and connections with others. These opportunities are especially important for young people with spina bifida, who may experience social isolation because of their disability.

Most young children's perceptions of friendship revolve around the sharing of toys, play materials, and enjoyable activities. For older children and especially adolescents, friendship takes on new meanings. The sharing of private thoughts and feelings grows more important. Children value respect and loyalty, and they increasingly develop an understanding of the interdependence of friends.

Feeling lonely from time to time is normal during childhood and adolescence. About one in ten of all children reports feeling lonely; undoubtedly, others also feel lonely but deny these feelings. Giving children opportunities to cultivate new friendships and offering support and advice can minimize this loneliness. We can all get by with a little help from our friends! Through our friends, we feel worthy and valued. Moreover, friends can help open doors to recreational experiences and the broader world outside.

LEISURE SKILLS AND RECREATIONAL OPPORTUNITIES

One of my favorite questions to ask families in clinic is, "What do you do for fun?" Sadly, the pressures of earning a living and keeping the family going often don't leave much time and energy for recreation. In recent years, however, I have been heartened by the number of families who are making recreation a priority. Not only are they enjoying a range of hobbies and adventures together, but they are also teaching their children a very valuable life lesson: playing is good for us!

Increasing recognition of the benefits of recreation has led to a mushrooming interest in leisure. Universities open new departments of leisure studies, magazines about crafts and computers appear on store shelves, and theme parks seem to spring up out of nowhere. Leisure is probably America's fastest growing industry!

For people with spina bifida, one of the exciting implications of this explosion is that recreational opportunities are more readily available to them now than ever before. Sometimes, the opportunities are there for the taking. More often, however, they have to be created with a lot of energy and enthusiasm. A young man with spina bifida and his father, who had always enjoyed fishing and hunting, worked hard to establish a sports club for outdoors enthusiasts with disabilities. The father has since died, but he has left behind greatly enhanced opportunities for others.

When it comes to sports, there is a range of possible involvement. Some like the more passive involvement of the spectator, whereas others like to participate actively in sports. Even following sports in the newspaper and on TV can be fun and rewarding. For those who want to play—and I think that children should be encouraged to do so—there are growing numbers of competitive sports from which to choose. Wheelchair tennis is very popular. In North Carolina and elsewhere in the United States, wheelchair basketball is the rage. The local team, named Wheels of Steel, has been a great source of enjoyment and pride for all involved. Such sports are played by a large age range; thus younger kids have role models, and the "seniors" can move on to provide a leadership role. On an international level, wheelchair racing is a seriously competitive sport, with some seriously committed athletes! The technology has undergone great advances in recent years. Racing chairs have a low seat, one large front tire, and lightweight, tubular frames. Athletes sit low in kneeling positions, hitting their wheel rims with enormously strong arms as they race.

As in all competitive sports, wheelchair sports carry some risk of injury. For safety, helmets should be used when racing or cycling on the road. It is advisable to build up gradually, because injuries from overuse of muscles are very common when taking up new sports. Those who take Ditropan should be careful to avoid excessive sun exposure, for they are prone to flushing and heatstroke. Also, there is a risk of skin injury, especially when the sport requires you to assume a different position or use special equipment; skin needs to be checked and rechecked!

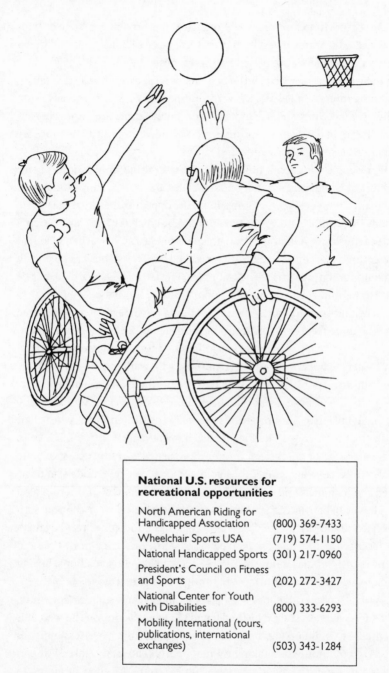

National U.S. resources for recreational opportunities

North American Riding for Handicapped Association	(800) 369-7433
Wheelchair Sports USA	(719) 574-1150
National Handicapped Sports	(301) 217-0960
President's Council on Fitness and Sports	(202) 272-3427
National Center for Youth with Disabilities	(800) 333-6293
Mobility International (tours, publications, international exchanges)	(503) 343-1284

Figure 11.4. A wide range of recreational opportunities is available for people of all ages with disabilities.

Of course, sport is only one kind of recreation. The arts can be life-affirming, giving an unparalleled opportunity for stimulation, expression, and communication. It is important to recognize the talents and affinities that children show: the child with a dramatic flair can then be steered toward a children's drama group at an early age, or a child with musical ability can begin to learn to play an instrument.

Other recreational opportunities for children with disabilities include Boy Scouts and Girl Scouts, bowling, and horseback riding. Even skiing and waterskiing are now readily accessible to people who use wheelchairs. A few resources are provided in Figure 11.4.

Finally, I must make an especially strong recommendation for the value of summer camps. Specialized camps for children with spina bifida provide a unique experience in self-reliance, social skills, and having fun without parents. When looking into camp opportunities, parents should find out about the experience of the staff, the staff-camper ratio, the nature of the accommodations, the accessibility of the camp, and how health care needs of the campers are met. The local chapter of the SBAA or an equivalent organization should be helpful in evaluating a prospective camp.

The family, education, work, and play: these things are the bedrock of our lives. As we grow up and develop, we must take on new challenges and set new goals for ourselves. Nobody's life story is free of trouble and pain. As my aerobics instructor says, "No pain, no gain!" But with effort, initiative, and a willingness to reach out for support and reach up to new opportunities, each of us creates something unique in life; and together, we make the world a better place. It is my hope that this book about spina bifida gives information and encouragement to many people whose lives are touched by this condition.

Directory of Spina Bifida Associations

U.S. SPINA BIFIDA ASSOCIATIONS

NATIONAL ORGANIZATION
Spina Bifida Association of America (SBAA), 4590 MacArthur Boulevard NW, Suite 250, Washington, DC 20007
Tel.: (202) 944-3285; Fax: (202) 944-3295
Web site: http://www.sbaa.org

ALABAMA
SBA of Alabama, P.O. Box 130538, Birmingham, AL 35213
Tel.: (205) 978-7287

ARIZONA
SBA of Arizona, 1001 East Fairmount, Phoenix, AZ 85014
Tel.: (602) 274-3323; Fax: (602) 274-7632
Web site: http://www.azspinabifida.org

ARKANSAS
SBA of Arkansas, P.O. Box 24663, Little Rock, AR 72221
Tel.: (501) 978-7222

CALIFORNIA
SBA of Greater San Diego, P.O. Box 232272, San Diego, CA 92193-2272
Tel.: (619) 491-9018; Fax: (619) 275-3361
Web site: http://www.spinabifidasandiego.org

SBA of Greater Rialto, 1014 W. Jackson St., Rialto, CA 92376
Tel.: (909) 875-1650; Fax: (909) 875-5437

COLORADO
SBA of Colorado, 4935 W. 28th Ave., Denver, CO 80212
Tel.: (720) 300-7502; Fax: (800) 544-1920
Web site: http://www.coloradospinabifida.org

CONNECTICUT

SBA of Connecticut, P.O. Box 2545, Hartford, CT 06146-2545
Tel.: (860) 704-0643; Fax: (860) 345-2600
Web site: http://www.sbac.org

DELAWARE

SBA of the Delaware Valley, P.O. Box 468, Media, PA 19063-0468
Tel.: (800) 223-0222 or (215) 676-8950; Fax: (610) 380-9304
Web site: http://www.sbadv.org

FLORIDA

SBA of Central Florida, P.O. Box 547970, Orlando, FL 32854-7970
Tel.: (407) 263-8350; Fax: (407) 862-8988
Web site: http://www.sbacf.org

SBA of Florida, 807 Children's Way, Jacksonville, FL 32207
Tel.: (800) 722-6355; Fax: (904) 390-3466
Web site: http://www.spinabifidafla.org

SBA of Florida Space Coast, 3685 Starlight Ave., Merritt Island, FL 32953
Tel.: (321) 454-9737; Fax: (321) 454-9737

SBA of Jacksonville, 807 Children's Way, Jacksonville, FL 32207
Tel.: (904) 390-3686; Fax: (904) 390-3466
Web site: http://www.sbaj.org

SBA of Southeast Florida, P.O. Box 15113, Plantation, FL 33318
Tel.: (954) 472-4089; Fax: (954) 472-7252

SBA of Tampa Bay, Inc., P.O. Box 151038, Tampa, FL 33684
Tel.: (813) 933-4827
Web site: http://lingming.tripod.com/sbatb/frames.html

GEORGIA

SBA of Georgia, 3355 NE Expressway #207, Atlanta, GA 30341
Tel.: (770) 454-7600; Fax: (770) 454-7678
Web site: http://www.spinabifidaofgeorgia.org

ILLINOIS

Illinois SBA, 3080 Ogden Ave. Suite 103, Lisle, IL 60532
Tel.: (630) 637-1050; Fax: (630) 637-1066
Web site: http://www.illinoisspinabifidaassociation.com/

INDIANA

SBA of Central Indiana, P.O. Box 19814, Indianapolis, IN 46219-0814
Tel.: (317) 592-1630; Fax: (317) 351-2010
Web site: http://www.sbaci.org

SBA of Northern Indiana, P.O. Box 2437, Elkhart, IN 46515
Tel.: (574) 293-4976

IOWA

SBA of Iowa, P.O. Box 1456, Des Moines, IA 50305
Tel.: (515) 964-8810

KANSAS

SBA of Kansas, P.O. Box 633, Wichita, KS 67201-0633
Tel.: (316) 516-7225

KENTUCKY

SBA of Kentucky, 982 Eastern Pkwy., Box 18, Louisville, KY 40217
Tel.: (502) 637-7363; Fax: (502) 637-1010
Web site: http://www.sbak.org

LOUISIANA

SBA of Greater New Orleans, P.O. Box 1346, Kenner, LA 70065
Tel.: (504) 737-5181; Fax: (504) 838-9046
Web site: http://www.sbagno.org

MARYLAND

Chesapeake-Potomac SBA; P.O. Box 1750, Annapolis, MD 21404
Tel.: (888) 733-0988; Fax: (410) 295-9744
Web site: http://www.chesapeakespinabifida.org

MASSACHUSETTS

Massachusetts SBA, 456 Lowell Street, Peabody, MA 01960
Tel.: (978) 531-6789

MICHIGAN

SBA of Southeastern Michigan, 12240 Woodcrest, Taylor, MI 48180
Tel.: (734) 287-3606; Fax: (734) 287-4043

SW Michigan SB and Hydrocephalus Association, P.O. Box 212, Mattawan,
MI 49071
Tel.: (269) 385-3959; Fax: (269) 342-9765

SBA of Upper Michigan, 1220 North 3rd St., Ishpeming, MI 49849
Tel.: (906) 485-5127
Web site: http://sba-up.8m.com

West Michigan SBA, 235 Wealthy Street SE, Grand Rapids, MI 49503
Tel.: (616) 392-1358
Web site: http://www.wmich.sba.tripod.com

MINNESOTA

SBA of Minnesota, P.O. Box 29323, Brooklyn Center, MN 55429
Tel.: (651) 228-0914; Fax: (651) 228-0914

MISSISSIPPI

SBA of Mississippi, 1511 Tracewood Dr., Jackson, MS 39211
Tel.: (601) 957-2410; Fax: (601) 957-2410
Web site: http://sbamiss.tripod.com

MISSOURI

SBA of Greater St. Louis, 5609 Hampton Ave., St. Louis, MO 63109-3435
Tel.: (800) 784-0983

NEBRASKA

SBA of Nebraska, 7101 Newport Ave. #206, Omaha, NE 68152-2151
Tel.: (402) 572-3570; Fax: (402) 572-3002
Web site: http://www.sban.info

NEW JERSEY

SBA of Bergen and Passaic Counties, 181 Glen Avenue, Midland Park, NJ 07432
Tel.: (201) 670-0590

SBA of the Tri-State Region, 84 Park Avenue, Flemington, NJ 08822
Tel.: (908) 782-7475; Fax: (908) 782-6102
Web site: http://www.sbatsr.org

NEW YORK

SBA of Albany/Capital District, 109 Spring Rd., Scotia, NY 12302
Tel.: (518) 399-9151
Web site: http://www.SBAAlbany.org

Greater Rochester SBA, P.O. Box 3, Fairport, NY 14450
Tel.: (585) 381-5471; Fax: (585) 264-9547

SBA of Nassau County, 218 White Ave., New Hyde Park, NY 11040
Tel.: (516) 354-4837

SBA of Western New York, P.O. Box 50, Williamsville, NY 14231-0050
Tel.: (716) 446-5595; Fax: (716) 735-7561

NORTH CAROLINA

SBA of North Carolina, 3915 Grace Court, Indian Trail, NC 28079
Tel.: (704) 893-0277; Fax: (704) 882-0988
Web site: http://www.sbanc.org

OHIO

SBA of Canton, P.O. Box 9089, Canton, OH 44711
Tel.: (330) 966-9208; Fax:(330) 863-1172

SBA of Cincinnati, 3245 Deborah Lane, Cincinnati, OH 45239
Tel.: (513) 923-1514
Web site: http://www.sbacincy.org

SBA of Greater Dayton, 6938 Wembley Circle, Centerville, OH 45459
Tel.: (937) 439-3830; Fax: (937) 434-4899
Web site: http://www.sbadayton.org

SBA of Northwest Ohio, 134 S. Findlay Park, P.O. Box 102, Portage, OH 43451
Tel.: (419) 686-2515

Tri-County SBA, P.O. Box 8701, Warren, OH 44484
Tel.: (330) 793-8544; Fax: (330) 793-8544

PENNSYLVANIA (*see also Delaware*)
SBA of Greater Pennsylvania, 209 East State Street, Suite B, Quarryville, PA 17566
Tel.: (717) 786-9280; Fax: (717)-786-8821
Web site: http://www.geocities.com/sbaofgpa

SBA of Greater Pittsburgh, 197 Bebout Rd., Venetia, PA 15367
Tel.: (724) 348-4286

RHODE ISLAND
SBA of Rhode Island, P.O. Box 6948, Warwick, RI 02887-6948
Tel.: (401) 732-7862; Fax: (401) 732-7862

TENNESSEE
SBA of Tennessee, 216 Sontag Drive, Franklin, TN 37064
Tel.: (615) 791-1518

TEXAS
Austin SBA, Inc., 9301 Bradner Drive, Austin, TX 78748
Tel.: (512) 292-6317; Fax: (512) 479-3845

SBA of Dallas, 705 West Ave. B, Suite 409, Garland, TX 75040
Tel.: (972) 238-8755; Fax: (972) 414-3772
Web site: http://www.sbdallas.org

SBA of Houston Gulf Coast, 624 Pasadena Blvd., Suite 305, Pasadena, TX 77506
Tel.: (281) 997-2378 or (713) 473-8035; Fax: (281) 997-2378
Web site: http://www.sbahgc.org

SBA of Texas, 2935 Thousand Oaks, Suite 6-124, San Antonio, TX 78247
Tel.: (210) 653-1800
Web site: http://www.sbatx.org

UTAH
SBA of Utah, P.O. Box 97, Bountiful, UT 84011-0097
Tel.: (801) 295-6558; Fax: (801) 451-2747
Web site: http://groups.yahoo.com/group/sbau

VIRGINIA
SBA of the Roanoke Valley, 1522 Muse Drive, Vinton, VA 24179
Tel.: (540) 890-1244

WASHINGTON
Evergreen SBA, P.O. Box 642, Sumner, WA 98390
Tel.: (253) 841-5717

WISCONSIN
SBA of Greater Fox Valley, 325 N. John St., Kimberly, WI 54136
Tel.: (920) 687-0801

SBA of Northern Wisconsin, P.O. Box 421, Schofield, WI 54476-0421
Tel.: (715) 359-9674

SBA of Wisconsin, 830 N. 109th Street, Suite 6, Wauwatosa, WI 53226
Tel.: (414) 607-9061; Fax: (414) 607-9602
Web site: http://sbawi.org

INTERNATIONAL SPINA BIFIDA ASSOCIATIONS

ARGENTINA
APEBI, Victor Hugo 1547, Capital Federal Republica Argentina
Tel.: 054 011 4568 1088; Fax: 054 011 4482 2282
Web site: http://www.apebi.org/

AUSTRALIA
Australian Spina Bifida and Hydrocephalus Association (ASBHA), P.O. Box 272
AU-Torrensville Plaza, SA 5031
Tel.: +61 8 8443 5200; Fax: +61 8 8443 5100
Web site: http://www.asbha.org.au

AUSTRIA
Spina Bifida und Hydrocephalus Österreich (SBHÖ), Postfach 88 A-1234 Vienna
Tel.: +43 664 492 0727; Fax: +43 1 879 2905

BELGIUM
Vereniging voor Spina Bifida en Hydrocephalus vzw (VSH), Drongenplein 26 B
9031 Drongen/Gent
Tel./Fax: +32 9 216 65 51
Web site: http://www.spinabifida.be

BRAZIL
Associação de Espinha Bifida e Hidrocefalia do Rio de Janiero (AEBH)
Tel.: +55 (21)2439 4550
Web site: http://www.aebh.kit.net

BULGARIA
Bulgarian Academy for Developmental Rehabilitation, at Dejstwije Slantschev
Latsch-Foundation, Blvd. Russki 117 4000, Plovdiv
Tel.: +359 32 270 872

BURUNDI
U.P.H.B., B.P. 536 Bujumbura
Tel.: 257 21 6273

CANADA
SB & H Association of Canada, 167—167 Lombard Avenue, Winnipeg, Manitoba
R3B OT6
Tel.: +1 204 925 3650

CHILE

Santiago SB & H Self-Help Group (ACHEB), Almirante Acevedo 5086 Vicatura, Santiago de Chile
Tel. +56 2 2635428

ACHAB, Sierra Blancha 7557 Las Condez, Santiago
Tel.: +56 2 224 2699

COLOMBIA

Colombia Fundación Mónica Uribe PorAmor, Carrera 77 # 33 a 73 Apt 402, Colombia

DENMARK

Rygmarvsbrokforeningen af 1988, Egebaeksvej 26 B, DK- 8270 Hoejbjerg
Web site: http://www.rygmarvsbrokforeningen.dk

ESTONIA

Seljaajusonga ja Vesipeahaigete Selts, Tervise 28, 13419, Tallinn
Tel.: +37 2 697 4239

FINLAND

Suomen CP-Liitto, Kaupintie 16 B FI-00440, Helsinki
Tel.: +358 9 5407 5414; Fax: +358 9 5407 5460
Web site: http://www.cp-liitto.fi

FRANCE

Fédération Française des Associations du Spina Bifida (FFASB), 58 rue du pré commun, 31230 L'ISLE en DODON France
Tel./Fax: +33 5 61 79 40 78
Web site: http://www.spinabifida.fr.st/

GERMANY

Arbeitsgemeinschaft Spina Bifida und Hydrocephalus (ASbH), Münsterstrasse 13, D-44145 Dortmund
Tel.: +49 231 86 1050-0; Fax: +49 231 86 1050-50
Web site: http://www.asbh.de

GREECE

c/o John C. Kouros, 3 Levido Str., N. Erythrea, P.O. Box 146 71 115 26, Athens

GUATEMALA

Asociación Guatemalteca de Espina Bifida (AGEB), 9a Av 46-63 Zona 12 Monte Maria 3, Ciudad de Guatemala
Tel.: (502) 477 3375; Fax: (502) 477 3375

HONDURAS

Farmacia Pineda Santa Barbara, 22101 Honduras

HONG KONG

The Childhood Spina Bifida Group of Hong Kong, Kwong Yau House, Room 805, Kwong Fuk Estate, Tai Po, NT, Hong Kong
Tel.: (852) 9163 4470

INDIA

Shantanu jindel, g-14 Krishna Marg c'sheme, Jaipur 302001

INDONESIA

Komunitas Spina Bifida Indonesia, JL. Mertilang XVIII KD 1/7, Sektor 9 Bintaro Jaya, Tangerang 15229
Web site: http://sb.blueviolin.com

IRELAND

Irish Association for Spina Bifida and Hydrocephalus, Old Nangor Road IE-Clondalkin, Dublin 22
Tel.: +353 1 457 2326; Fax: +353 1 457 2328

ITALY

Federazione Associazioni Italiane Spina Bifida e Idrocefalo (FAISBI), Via P. Chimer 35 I-250 17 Lonato (BS)
Tel.: +39 (0) 71 743594; Fax: +39 (0)71 202222
Web site: http://www.faisbi.cjb.net

JAPAN

Spina Bifida Association of Japan, 214 Ever Green Court 4-13-10, NakaRokugou Ota-ku, Tokyo
Tel.: +81 45 943 9079; Fax: +81 45 943 9145

KENYA

Kenya Association of Spina Bifida and Hydrocephalus, P.O. Box 30016, Nairobi

LUXEMBURG

Association pour le Spina Bifida, 5 Chemin de Bousberg Boîte Postale 20, L-7763 Bissen
Tel.: +352 859 188; Fax: +352 858 540

MALTA

c/o Mr. Lawrence Bezzina, 123 Cottoner Avenue FGURA PLA 17

MEXICO

c/o Mrs. Paulina Soto Morales, Alejandro Dumas #118, Jardine Vallarta CP 45020

The Mexican Association for Spina Bifida
Maurice Baring 295, Col. Jardines de la patria, Zapopan, Jalisco 45050
Tel./Fax: (55) 33 36 29 80 03

THE NETHERLANDS

BOSK Work Group Spina Bifida and Hydrocephalus, Postbus 3359, NL-3502 GJ Utrecht

Tel.: +31 30 2459090; Fax: +31 2313872
Web site: http://www.bosk.nl

NEW ZEALAND

Spina Bifida Support Group, P.O. Box 19281 Avondale, Auckland
Tel.: +64 9 4119261

NORWAY

Norwegian Association for Spina Bifida and Hydrocephalus, Pb 4568, Nydalen,
0404 OSLO
Web site: http://www.ryggmargsbrokk.org

PALESTINE

Abu Raya Rehabilitation Unit, Ramallh Jaffa St., P.O. Box 1424, Palestine

PERU

Asociación Peruana de Espina Bifida e Hidrocephalia Arequipa (APEBHI), Av
Jorge Chavez 527, Cerado Arequipa
Tel.: 054-206720

POLAND

Polish Association for Spina Bifida and Hydrocephalus (ASBP), ul. Żelazowej Woli
20/39a 20-853 Lublin
Tel./Fax: +48 081443 85 76

PORTUGAL

Associação Spina Bifida e Hidrocefalia de Portugal, Rua Botelho Vasconcelos Lote
567-D Zona-J Chelas, P-1900 Lisboa
Tel.: +351 185 9 6768 Fax: +351 1859 6768

ROMANIA

ASCHF Str. G-ral Haralambie nr. 36, 75208 Bucharest
Tel.: 402 3371875

SCOTLAND

Scottish Spina Bifida Association, 190 Queensferry Road, Edinburgh EH4 2BW
Tel.: +44 131 332 0743; Fax: +44 131 343 3651
Web site: http://www.ssba.org.uk

SOUTH AFRICA

Association for Spina Bifida and Hydrocephalus, 14 Avonwold Road
ZA-Saxonwold, 2196

SPAIN

Federación Española de Asociaciones de Espina Bifida e Hidrocefalia (FEAEBH),
Pechuan 14—Local 6, E-28002 Madrid
Tel.: +34 91 415 2013; Fax: +34 91 413 5845

Asociación de Padres con Hijos Espina Bifida (APHEB), Sorolla 10, Bloc B,
E-Barcelona 35
Tel.: +34 93 428 2180; Fax: +34 93 428 1934

SWEDEN

RBU, Box 6607, S-113 84 Stockholm

Tel.: +46 (0) 8 736 26 00; Fax: +46 (0) 8 30 14 10

SWITZERLAND

Geschäftsstelle SBH, Neuwiesenstrasse 11, CH-9034 Eggersriet

Tel.: +41 (0)71 877 28 54

TAIWAN

Tai-Tong Wong, MD N° 201, sec 2 Shih rd Tapei 11217

Tel./Fax: 886-2-8757587

TURKEY

Spina Bifida Dernegi Ege Universitesi Tip Fakultesi Cocuk Cerrahisi AD, T-35100 Bornova, Izmir

Tel.: +90 232 3881 412; Fax: +90 232 3422 142

Web site: http://alpha.med.ege.edu.tr/spina/

UGANDA

Cheshire Homes Kampala, P.O. Box 16548, Kampala

Tel.: 041 567410; Fax: 041 342729

UNITED KINGDOM

Association for Spina Bifida and Hydrocephalus (ASBAH), 42 Park Road, GB-Peterborough PE1 2UQ

Tel.: +44 1733 555988; Fax: +44 1733 555985

Web site: http://www.asbah.demon.co.uk/

VENEZUELA

Asociación Venezolana de la Espina Bifida (AVEB), Apart. Post. 88097 T.C. Hipico, Caracas, D.F.

Tel.: +582 693 1002 & 662 1681; Fax: +582 6936 154

References and Suggestions
for Further Reading

General

Bannister, C., and B. Tew, eds. (1991). *Current concepts in spina bifida and hydrocephalus*. London: MacKeith.

Hunt, G. (1990). Open spina bifida: Outcome for a complete cohort treated unselectively and followed into adulthood. *Developmental Medicine and Child Neurology* 32:108–18.

Klein, S. D. (1993). The challenge of communicating with parents. *Journal of Developmental and Behavioral Pediatrics* 14:184–91.

Lorber, J. (1971). Results of treatment of myelomeningocele. *Developmental Medicine and Child Neurology* 13:279–303.

Lorber, J. (1972). Spina bifida cystica: Results of treatment of 270 consecutive cases with criteria for selection for the future. *Archives of Diseases in Childhood* 47:854–73.

McLone, D. G. (1992). Continuing concepts in the management of spina bifida. *Pediatric Neurosurgery* 18:254–56.

Rowley-Kelly, F. L., and D. H. Reigel. (1993). *Teaching the child with spina bifida*. Baltimore: Paul H. Brookes.

Shurtleff, D. B., ed. (1986). *Myelodysplasias and extrophies: Significance, prevention, and treatment*. Orlando: Grune and Stratton.

World Health Organization. (1980). *International classification of impairments, disabilities, and handicaps*. Geneva, Switzerland: WHO.

Epidemiology

Czeizel, A. E., and I. Dudas. (1992). Prevention of the first occurrence of neural tube defects by periconceptional vitamin supplementation. *New England Journal of Medicine* 327:1832–35.

Greene, W. B., R. C. Terry, R. A. DeMai, and R. T. Herrington. (1991). Effect of race and gender on neurologic level in myelomeningocele. *Developmental Medicine and Child Neurology* 33:110–17.

Milunsky, A., H. Jick, S. Jick, C. L. Bruell, D. S. MacLaughlin, K. J. Rothman, and W. Willett. (1989). Multivitamin/folic acid supplementation in early pregnancy reduces the prevalence of neural tube defects. *Journal of the American Medical Association* 262:2847-52.

MRC Vitamin Study Research Group. (1991). Prevention of neural tube defects: Results of the Medical Research Council Vitamin Study. *Lancet* 338:131-37.

Mulinare, J., J. F. Cordero, J. D. Erickson, and R. J. Berry. (1988). Periconceptional use of multivitamins and the occurrence of neural tube defects. *Journal of the American Medical Association* 260:3141-45.

Sandford, M. K., G. E. Kissling, and P. E. Joubert. (1992). Neural tube defect etiology: New evidence concerning maternal hyperthermia, health, and diet. *Developmental Medicine and Child Neurology* 34:661-75.

Smithells, D. (1991). Prevention of spina bifida and hydrocephalus. In *Current concepts in spina bifida and hydrocephalus*, ed. C. Bannister and B. Tew, 1-15. London: MacKeith.

Cesarian Section

Luthy, D. A., T. Wardinsky, D. B. Shurtleff, D. E. Hickok, K. A. Hollenbach, and T. J. Benedetti. (1991). Cesarian section before onset of labor for babies with myelomeningocele. *New England Journal of Medicine* 324:662-66.

Screening Programs

Brock, D. J. H., and R. G. Sutcliffe. (1972). Alpha-fetoprotein in the antenatal diagnosis of anencephaly and spina bifida. *Lancet* 2:197-99.

Shurtleff, D. B. (1986). Prenatal diagnosis: Prevention and management for improved pregnancy outcome. In *Myelodysplasias and extrophies: Significance, prevention, and treatment*, ed. D. B. Shurtleff, 65-87. Orlando: Grune and Stratton.

Genetics and Embryology

Desmond, M. E. (1982). Description of the occlusion of the spinal cord lumen in early human embryos. *Anatomical Record* 204:89-93.

Seller, M. J. (1987). Neural tube defects and sex ratios. *American Journal of Medical Genetics* 26:699-707.

Myelomeningocele Repair/Chiari/Neurosurgery

Charney, E. B., J. B. Melchionni, and D. L. Antonucci. (1991). Ventriculitis in newborns with myelomeningocele. *American Journal of Diseases in Children* 145:287-90.

Dahl, M., G. Ahlsten, H. Carlson, and E. Ronne-Engström. (1995). Neurologic dysfunction above the cele level in children with spina bifida cystica: A prospective study to three years. *Developmental Medicine and Child Neurology* 37: 30-40.

McEnery, G., M. Borzyskowski, and T. C. S. Cox. (1992). The spinal cord in neurologically stable spina bifida: A clinical and MRI study. *Developmental Medicine and Child Neurology* 34:342–47.

McLone, D. G., and P. A. Knepper. (1989). The cause of Chiari II malformation: A unified theory. *Pediatric Neuroscience* 15:1–12.

McLone, D. G., D. Czyzewski, A. Raimondi, and R. Sommers. (1982). Central nervous system infections as a limiting factor in the intelligence of children with myelomeningocele. *Pediatrics* 70:338–42.

Moss, S. M., R. J. Marchbanks, and D. M. Burge. (1991). Long-term assessment of intracranial pressure using the tympanic membrane displacement measurement technique. *European Journal of Pediatric Surgery* 1 (Supplement): 25–26.

Piatt, J. H. (1992). Physical examination of patients with cerebrospinal fluid shunts: Is there useful information in pumping the shunt? *Pediatrics* 89:470–73.

Reigel, D. H. (1983). Tethered spinal cord. *Concepts in Pediatric Neurosurgery* 4:142–64.

Shurtleff, D. B., and J. T. Stuntz. (1986). Back closure. In *Myelodysplasias and extrophies: Significance, prevention, and treatment,* ed. D. B. Shurtleff, 117–50. Orlando: Grune and Stratton.

Urological Issues

Bauer, S. B., M. Hallett, S. Khoshbin, R. L. Lebowitz, K. R. Winston, S. Gibson, A. H. Colodny, and A. R. Retik. (1984). Predictive value of urodynamic evaluation in newborns with myelodysplasia. *Journal of the American Medical Association* 252:650–52.

Boone, T., C. Roehrborn, and G. Hurt. (1992). Transurethral electrotherapy for neurogenic bladder dysfunction in children with myelodysplasia: A prospective, randomized clinical trial. *Journal of Urology* 148:550–54.

Dector, R., P. Snyder, and T. Rosvanis. (1992). Transurethral electrical bladder stimulation. *Journal of Urology* 149:651–53.

Gross, A. J., F. Godeman, T. Michael, K. Weigle, and H. Huland. (1993). Urological findings in patients with neurosurgically treated tethered spinal cord. *Journal of Urology* 149:1510–11.

Joseph, D. B., S. B. Bauer, A. H. Colodny, J. Mandell, and A. B. Retik. (1989). Clean, intermittent catheterization of infants with neurogenic bladder. *Pediatrics* 84:78–82.

Kass, E. J., S. A. Koff, and A. C. Diokno. (1981). Fate of vesicoureteral reflux in children with myelodysplasia. *Journal of Urology* 125:63–69.

Lapides, J., A. C. Diokno, S. J. Silber, and B. S. Lowe. (1971). Clean intermittent self-catheterization in the treatment of urinary tract disease. *Journal of Urology* 107:458–63.

Sackett, C. K. (1993). Spina bifida: Implication for bladder and bowel management. *Urological Nursing* 13:104–6.

Schlager, T. A., S. Dilks, J. Trudell, T. S. Whittam, and J. O. Hendley. (1995). Bacteriuria in children with neurogenic bladder treated with intermittent catheterization: Natural history. *Journal of Pediatrics* 126:490–95.

Orthopedic Issues

Dudgeon, B. J., K. M. Jaff, and D. B. Shurtleff. (1991). Variations in midlumbar myelomeningocele: Implications for ambulation. *Pediatric Physical Therapy* 14:57–62.

Harris, M. B., and J. V. Banta. (1990). Cost of skin care in the myelomeningocele population. *Journal of Pediatric Orthopedics* 10:355–61.

Liptak, G. S., D. B. Shurtleff, J. W. Bloss, E. Baltus-Hebert, and P. Manitta. (1992). Mobility aids for children with high-level myelomeningocele: Parapodium versus wheelchair. *Developmental Medicine and Child Neurology* 34:787–96.

Mazur, J. M., M. B. Menelaus, D. R. V. Dickens, and W. G. Doig. (1986). Efficacy of surgical management for scoliosis in myelomeningocele: Correction of deformity and alteration of functional status. *Journal of Pediatric Orthopedics* 6: 568–75.

Mazur, J. M., D. B. Shurtleff, M. B. Menelaus, and J. Colliver. (1989). Orthopedic management of high-level spina bifida: Early walking compared with early use of a wheelchair. *Journal of Bone and Joint Surgery* 71-A:56–61.

Menelaus, M. B. (1980). *The orthopedic management of spina bifida cystica.* Edinburgh: Churchill Livingstone.

Rosenstein, B. D., W. B. Greene, R. T. Herrington, and A. S. Blum. (1987). Bone density in myelomeningocele: The effects of ambulatory status and other factors. *Developmental Medicine and Child Neurology* 29:486–94.

Growth

Greene, S. A., M. Frank, M. Zachmann, and M. Prader. (1985). Growth and sexual development in children with myelomeningocele. *European Journal of Pediatrics* 144:146–48.

Rotenstein, D., D. H. Reigel, and L. L. Flom. (1989). Growth hormone treatment accelerates growth of short children with neural tube defects. *Journal of Pediatrics* 115:417–20.

Latex Allergy

Leger, R. R., and E. Meerapol. (1992). Children at risk: Latex allergy and spina bifida. *Journal of Pediatric Nursing* 7:371–76.

Early Intervention

Mazur, J. M., M. B. Menelaus, I. Hudson, and A. Stillwell. (1986). Hand function in patients with spina bifida cystica. *Journal of Pediatric Orthopedics* 6:442–47.

Williamson, G. G., ed. (1987). *Children with spina bifida: Early intervention*. Baltimore: Paul H. Brookes.

Effects on Learning/Psychological Issues

Friedrich, W. N., M. C. Lovejoy, J. Shaffer, D. B. Shurtleff, and R. L. Beilke. (1991). Cognitive abilities and achievement status of children with myelomeningocele: A contemporary sample. *Journal of Pediatric Psychology* 16:423–28.

Lavigne, J. V., D. Nolan, and D. G. McLone. (1988). Temperament, coping, and psychological adjustment in young children with myelomeningocele. *Journal of Pediatric Psychology* 13:363–78.

Lollar, D. J. (1990). Learning patterns among spina bifida children. *Zeitschrift für Kinderchirurgie* 45:39.

Sandler, A. D. (1989). Social development in middle childhood. *Pediatric Annals* 18:380–87.

Tew, B. (1991). The effects of spina bifida and hydrocephalus upon learning and behavior. In *Current concepts in spina bifida and hydrocephalus*, ed. C. Bannister and B. Tew, 158–79. London: MacKeith.

Wallander, J. L., W. S. Feldman, and J. W. Varni. (1989). Physical status and psychosocial adjustment in children with spina bifida. *Journal of Pediatric Psychology* 14:89–102.

Adolescent/Adult Health Care Issues

Blum, R. W. (1983). The adolescent with spina bifida. *Clinical Pediatrics* 22:331–34.

Börjeson, M. C., and J. Lagergren. (1990). Life conditions of adolescents with myelomeningocele. *Developmental Medicine and Child Neurology* 32:698–706.

Hayden, P. W., S. L. H. Davenport, and M. M. Campbell. (1979). Adolescents with myelodysplasia: Impact of physical disability on emotional maturation. *Pediatrics* 64:53–59.

Hunt, G. M., and A. Poulton. (1995). Open spina bifida: A complete cohort reviewed 25 years after closure. *Developmental Medicine and Child Neurology* 37:19–29.

Lollar, D. J., ed. (1994). *Preventing secondary conditions associated with spina bifida or cerebral palsy*. Washington, D.C.: Spina Bifida Association of America.

McLone, D. G. (1989). Spina bifida today: Problems adults face. *Seminars in Neurology* 9:169–75.

Rauen, K. K., and E. J. Aubert. (1992). A brighter future for adults who have myelomeningocele—one form of spina bifida. *Orthopedic Nursing* 11:16–25.

Sexuality

Edser, P., and G. Ward. (1991). Sexuality, sex, and spina bifida. In *Current concepts in spina bifida and hydrocephalus*, ed. C. Bannister and B. Tew, 202–11. London: MacKeith.

Sandler, A. D., G. Worley, E. C. Leroy, S. D. Stanley, and S. Kalman. (1994). Sexual knowledge and experience among young men with spina bifida. *European Journal of Pediatric Surgery* 4 (Supplement 1): 36–37.

Sandler, A. D., G. Worley, E. C. Leroy, S. D. Stanley, and S. Kalman. (1996). Sexual function and erection capability in young men with spina bifida. *Developmental Medicine and Child Neurology* 38:823–29.

Sloan, S. L. (1993). *Sexuality issues in spina bifida*. Washington, D.C.: Spina Bifida Association of America.

Sloan, S. L. (1994). *Sexuality and the person with spina bifida*. Washington, D.C.: Spina Bifida Association of America.

Family Issues

Carr, J. (1991). The effect of neural tube defects on the family and its social functioning. In *Current concepts in spina bifida and hydrocephalus*, ed. C. Bannister and B. Tew, 180–92. London: MacKeith.

Kazak, A. E., and M. Williams-Clark. (1986). Stress in families of children with myelomeningocele. *Developmental Medicine and Child Neurology* 28:220–28.

McCormick, M. C., E. B. Charney, and M. M. Stemmler. (1986). Assessing the impact of a child with spina bifida on the family. *Developmental Medicine and Child Neurology* 28:53–61.

Spaulding, B. R., and S. B. Morgan. (1986). Spina bifida children and their parents: A population prone to family dysfunction? *Journal of Pediatric Psychology* 11:359–74.

Tew, B., H. Payne, and K. M. Laurence. (1974). Must a family with a handicapped child be a handicapped family? *Developmental Medicine and Child Neurology* 16 (Supplement 32): 95–98.

Employment and Financial Issues

American Council on Education. (1992). *Transition Resource Guide*. HEATH Resource Center. Washington, D.C.: U.S. Department of Education.

Equal Employment Opportunity Commission. (1991). *The Americans with Disabilities Act: Your employment rights as an individual with a disability*. Washington, D.C.: EEOC.

National Information Center for Children and Youth with Disabilities. (1991). *Transition Summary*. Washington, D.C.: U.S. Department of Education.

Rosenfeld, L. R. (1994). *Your child and health care: A "dollars and sense" guide for families with special needs*. Baltimore: Paul H. Brookes.

Schlachter, G. A., and R. D. Webb. (1995). *Financial aid for the disabled and their families, 1995–1996*. Redwood City, Calif.: Reference Service Press.

Worley, G., L. R. Rosenfeld, and J. Lipscomb. (1991). Financial counseling for families of children with spina bifida. *Developmental Medicine and Child Neurology* 33:679–89.

Index

Adult outcomes, 3
Advocacy, 214–15, 228–29
Agent Orange, 35
Alpha-fetoprotein, 6, 36–38
Americans with Disabilities Act (ADA), xiii,
191, 194, 236–38
Amniocentesis, 37, 44
Anencephaly, 17
Antibiotics, 58, 65, 70, 176–77
Anticholinergic medications, 71, 73, 162–64
Apnea, 67
Arnold-Chiari II malformation. *See* Chiari
malformation
Ataxia, 112, 202
Attention deficit, 132, 154–56; medications
for, 156. *See also* Learning disabilities
Autonomic nerves, 22

Biofeedback, 168
Bisacodyl, 169–70
Bladder augmentation procedures, 166
Bladder dysfunction, 24–25, 71–73, 159,
162; and open bladder neck, 164, 166.
See also Anticholinergic medications;
Catheterization, clean intermittent;
Continence
Bladder stimulation, 168
Bowel dysfunction, 26, 168–70. *See also*
Constipation
Braces, 86–92, 135–36; purposes of, 86;
standing frame, 87–88; parapodium, 88;
swivel walkers, 88–89; reciprocating gait
orthosis, 89–90; HKAFO, 90; KAFO, 90;
AFO, 91; independent use of, 124–25; for
scoliosis, 182

Camp, 206, 241
Casting, 108, 136
Catheterization, clean intermittent,
71–73, 159–67; equipment for, 160–
61; procedure, 161–62; teaching self-
catheterization, 166–67
Centers for Disease Control (CDC), 3, 34,
138
Central nervous system, 11
Cerebrospinal fluid (CSF), 16, 111, 201–2.
See also Hydrocephalus
Cesarian section, 45–46
Chiari malformation: embryology of, 12–
14; and feeding difficulties, 56, 111–13;
and Chiari crisis in newborn, 67–70;
and clinical-pathologic findings, 68;
assessment and treatment of, 68–69;
symptoms of, 112, 202
Clubfoot, 136–38
Cognitive abilities. *See* Development:
cognitive; Learning disabilities
Communication between parents and
professionals, xiv, 48–49, 82–83
Compliance, 204–5
Constipation, 102–4; and dietary treatment, 103–4; and laxatives, 104, 169; and
continence, 168, 170
Continence: and toilet training, 101; and
independence, 159; and medications,
162–64; persistent urinary incontinence,
164–66; ostomy, 166; surgical treatments, 166; and bladder stimulation,
168; and bowel programs, 168–70. *See
also* Catheterization, clean intermittent
Contraception, 192